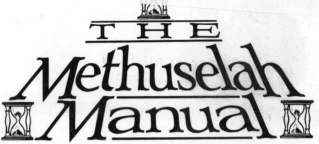

THE Methuselah Manual

The 3% Formula for Staying Young, Healthy and Sexy

DR. DAVID C. GARDNER

DR. GRACE JOELY BEATTY

AMERICAN TRAINING AND RESEARCH ASSOCIATES, INC., PUBLISHERS
P.O. Box 118, Windham, New Hampshire 03087

i

Illustrations and cover design by Deirdre McCullough Grunwald
Cover logo by H. Michael McCullough
Cover photograph by Jerry Glickman
Composition by Fish & Maria Design Associates, Lawrence, MA 01841
Printed by Boyd Printing Company, Inc., Albany, NY 12210

First Edition

Library of Congress Cataloging in Publication Data
Gardner, David C..
    The Methuselah Manual: The 3% Formula for Staying Young, Healthy and Sexy
    Includes Bibliography, Index
    1. Longevity. 2.Psychology - Popular Works. 3. Hygiene. 4. Medicine, preventive. I. Beatty, Grace Joely, joint author.
    II. Title
    Library of Congress Catalog Number: 84-72980

ISBN: 0-961-39999-6

ACKNOWLEDGMENTS

2273636

In any project of this scope there is always one person who makes things come together, who anticipates the problems and finds ways to solve them, who cheers everybody up when the tensions become intolerable and who helps bring reality and balance to the overworked crew. *The Methuselah Manual* project was most fortunate to have had its own special person who did all these things and more. We want to thank Jo Anne Schottler from the bottom of our hearts for giving so much of herself to keep the project and the authors running smoothly. We also want to thank her husband, Fred, and her children, Dawn and Jeffrey, for allowing us to steal some of her time from them.

Choosing an artist to interact with us under the pressure of many deadlines was risky business. We followed our instincts and asked Deirdre McCullough Grunwald to illustrate our text. Our instincts were correct. We found a gold mine of talent overlayed with a calming sense of proportion, sound ideas and a willingness to go beyond the call of duty to meet a genuinely unrealistic time schedule. Thank you, Deirdre, for sharing your wonderful talent and time with us!

This is the first book we have written on computers. In the beginning we were faced with a nightmare of strange commands and terms like "control C" and "floppy discs." We had to learn how to use the system quickly and to keep our heads when things went wrong. We lived on the verge of panic until Elizabeth Ross came to our rescue. Liz, we thank you for your patience and all your help. We don't know how we could have made the deadlines without you.

We want to acknowledge our families, friends, professional colleagues and business associates who gave so freely of their time in reading all or part of the manuscript and giving us helpful suggestions and comments: Joseph Beatty, Shirley Beatty, Linda Beatty, Carol Bumgardner, William R. Bumgardner, J.D., Reverend Richard Burke, Joseph "Barney" Campiola, Jack T. Evjy, M.D., Sheila Evjy, R.N., Jerome T. Glickman, Ed. D., Jeanne Mattie, William Patenaude, Arthur C. Provencal, D.C., Bonnie Putnam, Gerry Putnam, Henry Quellmalz, Fred Schottler and Lester "Tommy" Thompson. We would also like to acknowledge the efforts of Jennifer Robin Beatty, David Sauer, Dawn "Sunrise" Schottler and Margaret Gunning. We also want to thank Joshua and Jessica for their patience.

Last but not least, we want to acknowledge our indebtedness to all the physical and social scientists and scholars whose research efforts have contributed to the current scientific knowledge and understanding about how human beings live, work, think, love, learn and grow old gracefully.

D.C.G.
G.J.B.

PREFACE

Although we didn't know it at the time, *The Methuselah Manual* began the day we decided to accept full responsibility for our own mental and physical well-being. We bought bikes, cleaned the processed food out of our kitchen and began trying to modify our own behavior so we could learn to exercise, cook, eat and relax in ways that would increase our vitality and youthfulness.

We read all the popular literature on how to prevent illness and maintain vigorous health through nutrition, exercise, yoga and meditation. We discovered that two essential elements were missing. First, the psychological aspects of life extension were either ignored or given only lip service. Second, we discovered that none of the books was truly holistic in its approach. While most gave good advice, the emphasis was usually on a single approach to improving life. This meant that we had to read a great many books to get a complete picture of the things we had to do to improve our lives.

Thus, out of our own frustration in acquiring and applying preventive health care information, the idea for *The Methuselah Manual* was born. *The Methuselah Manual* is designed to be read quickly, in small bits and pieces, as you have time in your busy schedule. It contains all the information that a person just getting interested in life extension and preventive health care will need to make immediate and permanent changes in his or her life. For those who have read extensively on the subject but haven't had much success in making permanent changes, it offers easy-to-follow instructions on behavior modification. Because of our readability goal, there are no footnotes or quotations. The facts in this book are based on published research, and for those who want to read in depth, there is an extensive list of references to both scientific and popular literature at the back of this book.

We are trained researchers in the behavioral sciences and have published numerous research articles. We train doctoral candidates in the behavioral sciences to do research and have written a textbook on how to do it. However, we are not medical researchers and therefore have had to rely on the research of others in areas of this book where we are not experts. We gratefully acknowledge all those who have published scientific research and clinical findings which have helped us to make this book as up to date and as comprehensive as possible.

Caution: The information in this book is educational in nature and should not be used as a substitute for sound medical and psychological care. We want to stress the importance of following the advice of your physician, psychologist or nutritionist as related to possible personal use of any of the information in this book. Do not ignore the specific warnings in the chapters on aerobics, flexibility, fasting and food supplements.

AD ASTRA PER ASPERA

CONTENTS

SECTION TWO
PSYCHOLOGY OF RELAXATION AND STRESS PREVENTION

SECTION THREE
THE PSYCHOLOGY OF PHYSICAL FITNESS

SECTION FOUR
THE PSYCHOLOGY OF CONTROLLING
YOUR BODY CHEMISTRY

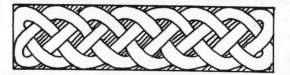

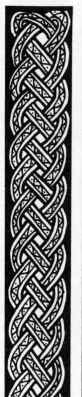
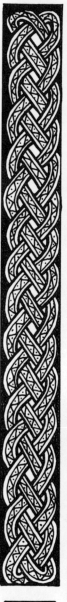

SECTION ONE

The Psychology Of Longevity

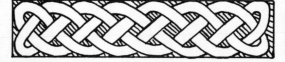

CHAPTER ONE

What Can This Book Do For Me?

Can I Really Improve the Quality and Length of My Life?

The answer is *yes, if you decide to do something about taking care of yourself.*

There is a vast amount of scientific information that can help you make your life healthier, help you look and feel younger and help you increase your self-confidence and energy level.

The key to improving your life is not simply finding out what to do. The real key is in learning how to permanently modify your own behaviors so that you can use the knowledge that is already available.

This Book Is About Change

Although aging is inevitable, getting old is related to mental and physical factors present in your lifestyle that *are under your control.* However, you must be prepared to make some changes in your life. If you insist on doing exactly what you have always done, be prepared to live the length and quality of life of the average American. If you want more than just the average, this book can help you make the necessary

Staying young is related to factors under your control.

changes. As you make your plans to go forward into something new, it is a good idea to have some benchmarks to help you check your progress. This book will help you establish those benchmarks.

While the status of your physical health is extremely important in trying to assess where you should begin your nutritional and exercise progam to stay young, healthy and sexy, it is actually fruitless to begin without making a psychological assessment of your readiness to follow through on a program which will require you to make changes in the way you live. This book will help you address the following problems:

1. ALL HUMAN BEINGS RESIST CHANGE

Although other health, diet and life extension books may offer good advice, they don't tell you how to make the changes so that they become a permanent part of your way of doing things. You need to learn how to overcome your normal resistance. In order to do this, you need to acquire a basic understanding of the principles of self-behavior modification so that you can apply these principles to your own situation. This book gives you step-by-step illustrations of those principles and tells you how to implement them.

2. IT AIN'T EASY!

What all the other books don't tell you is that making these changes is not easy. In fact the typical case goes like this:

Typical Case

Bernie knew he was in trouble when he began puffing every time he walked up the flight of stairs to his neighbor's front porch. One day, on his way to work, he suffered a major heart attack. After surgery, during recovery and at periodic intervals thereafter, his physician attempted to get him to change his diet, begin an exercise program and give up smoking. His father had died of a heart attack at age 50. Bernie was 45, looked 65, smoked, ate a diet heavily laden with red meat and fat and little or no fiber. Because of his wife's constant nagging he quit smoking for three days. Then he switched to low-tar cigarettes, rationalizing that it was better than the "pressure" he felt when not smoking. He switched from hard liquor to beer. Several years later he was back in the hospital for a triple bypass. Bernie, obviously, doesn't know how to learn from his experiences. He doesn't have a long-life personality. He could add years to his life by teaching himself to behave in a self-benefiting way.

We believe science offers us a way to prevent premature aging and death from the modern-society diseases of cancer, heart problems, diabetes and the like. These diseases stem from the stress imposed on us by our hard-driving culture, the breakdown of supportive social structures, the evolution of a fat- and sugar-oriented diet, the fast-food syndrome and the chemical nightmare called modern industrial progress, which has filled our everyday environment with toxic chemicals.

WHAT WE BELIEVE

Our thesis is that all the biological approaches to life extension, from exercise programs to the latest biochemical supplements to semi-starvation, are very likely to be totally ineffective for many of the people who buy or read the books or articles on the topic. Too many of the readers simply are unable to make the necessary permanent changes in their diet and lifestyle because they lack the knowledge of how to modify and control their own behavior. So instead of changing, they buy the next book or magazine...looking, searching for the "right" answers...not realizing that the first thing they must do is learn how to modify their own behavior. We also believe that as of this moment the behavioral and physical sciences have provided us with the information to enable you to increase your chances of living a life that is healthy both psychologically and physically. Such a life would not focus on adding years to your life but on adding life to your years, however many there are!

Throughout this book we will stress the importance of how your personality, your beliefs and your expectations are directly related to your health and thus your chances of staying young, healthy and sexy. There is a growing body of social-science research that continually points to the often-underestimated or ignored role that psychological well-being has in preventing your early demise.

Your psychological well-being plays an important role in longevity.

What Is A Long-Life Personality?

There are many people who believe that living a long life automatically means learning to live a boring life, that is, giving up the excitement of their present lifestyle. They think, "I have too much going on in my life. There is too much stress, but I like it the way it is. There are too many things I want to accomplish before I die. I have neither the time nor the inclination to sit on the front porch and watch the world go by in order to add years to my life. I'm not ready to go out to pasture. Besides, I wouldn't be able to live long under those conditions because I'd die of boredom!" People who think like that are wrong.

Can you guess which group of Americans lives the longest? It is the people who are listed in Who's Who. Since we can assume that these are achievement oriented people who have a great deal going on in their lives and who deal with stress all the time, we can negate the idea of the rocking-chair approach to long life. In fact, many studies demonstrate that people who retire with nothing to do and nothing to look forward to die relatively quickly.

Which group of Americans lives longest?

Regardless of whether they are listed in Who's Who, a person with a long-life personality is a person who deals well with change and is able to maintain a lifestyle that is beneficial to his or her mental and physical health. If you have a long-life personality you have the following skills and abilities:

Characteristics Of A Long-Life Personality

---

1. YOU ACCEPT RESPONSIBILITY FOR YOUR OWN ACTIONS

This includes a belief or recognition that responsibility for your own mental and physical well-being rests squarely on your own shoulders. In our method of teaching you how to make changes in your life-style, the degree to which you accept or can learn to accept the responsibility for your own life is the foundation upon which everything else is built.

2. YOU KNOW HOW TO SET GOALS, TO MAKE COMMITMENTS, TO FOLLOW THROUGH AND "EXPECT" TO SUCCEED

This involves not only setting your own goals but also using the power of goals and

7

expectancies that others may have for you. This book will teach you how to set goals and give you a way of following through on those goals.

3. **YOU KNOW HOW TO MAKE PERMANENT MODIFICATIONS IN YOUR OWN BEHAVIOR**

The overall theme of this book is to help you learn how to modify your own behaviors as they relate to your own well-being.

4. **YOU KNOW HOW TO RELAX AND DEAL EFFECTIVELY WITH STRESS** Using this relaxed state (sometimes called the alpha state) you can use visualization and positive statements to help improve your performance and achieve personal goals more efficiently.

The wonderful thing about all of these characteristics is that they are not predetermined at birth. They are learned characteristics that can be acquired at any time during your life. If you don't already have them, this book will help you acquire them.

What Is The 3% Formula?

Simply put, the 3% formula is the portion of your total time that you will have to devote to yourself each week to stay young, healthy and sexy. Three percent of the 168 hours in a week amounts to a total of five hours per week, or approximately 45 minutes per day. This is only a little more than the time you would spend watching a half-hour television program every night. It does require an investment of your time, but it is the best investment you will ever make. The decision to make the investment, however, is yours. No one else can make it for you.

The 3% formula is 3% of your total time per week.

The formula uses only hours devoted to new learnings or habits that you will have to acquire and maintain. It does not include initial start-up time or old learnings or tasks for which you will substitute new ways of doing things. For example, if you are not now aerobically exercising, then the time devoted to this will be part of the 3% formula when you add this as a new habit.

However, time spent shopping for healthier foods is simply substituted for time spent shopping for less desirable foodstuffs; therefore, you don't count this as additional time in your schedule. You have to shop. You have to cook. You have to eat. You have to deal with your job, your boss or business partner, your loved ones, your friends, etc. right now. If you acquire a long-life personality, you will be dealing with these situations and people differently, but the time spent will be more beneficial and effective. Therefore a modification of time you would normally spend anyway is not considered part of the 3% formula. In fact, when you master some of the techniques presented in this book, you may have to spend less of your personal time dealing with interpersonal problems and can devote more of your own time to things you want to do to stay happy! So let's add it up by looking at Dave's 3% profile:

THE 3% FORMULA
Example of Dave's Time Commitment
Minimum Weekly Program

New Habit Acquired	Permanent Time Added to Schedule per Week
Cooking Healthy Food (versus old way)	No Additional Time

THE 3% FORMULA
Minimum Weekly Program, continued

New Habit Acquired	Permanent Time Added to Schedule per Week
Shopping for Healthy Food (versus old way)	No Additional Time
Handling Loved Ones in Less Stressful Manner (versus old way)	No Additional Time
Handling Social Problems in Less Stressful Manner (versus old way)	No Additional Time
Handling Work Problems in Less Stressful Manner (versus old way)	No Additional Time
Self-Directed Stress-Reduction Program (Meditation)	2 hrs. per week (20 min. per day, 6 days per week)
Aerobic Fitness Program	1⅓ hrs. per week (20 min. per day, 4 days per week)
Flexibility Fitness Program	1⅔ hrs. per week (20 min. per day, 5 days per week)
	Total New Hours = 5

One important thing to remember about the 3% formula is that you do not have to limit yourself to five hours per week of aerobics, relaxation and flexibility training. If you desire, you can spend more time, particularly with your flexibility program, and gain additional benefits.

How Do I Use This Book?

The *Methuselah Manual* contains easy-to-understand, step-by-step directions for developing a long-life personality and lifestyle. The book is organized so that you can easily acquire new and more effective ways to deal with your home, work and social environment. In addition, The *Methuselah Manual* offers a low-key approach to acquiring ways to keep your body fit and flexible, to control your body chemistry and to learn how to really relax.

After reading this first section you don't have to read the book in any order. For example, if you feel you want to make your first attempt at changing to a healthy lifestyle in the nutrition area, then that is where you should begin. Once completed, you can then branch out into aerobics or flexibility or interpersonal skills. A number of chapters include final pages where you can write your goals and make notes. You can also make notes in the right column of any page.

After reading the first section, you can read the book in any order.

Write your notes in the margins and on note pages at the end of each chapter.

The chart below shows you what each chapter has to offer. Your final program must include at least one of the major activities in each section (e.g., aerobics, better diet, etc.) but take your time. Don't turn your long-life program into a stressful event.

The Long-Life Personality and Lifestyle Program

Program Goal	Section	Chapter No.
1. Develop an understanding of the long-life personality. Learn how to modify your behavior so you can stay young, healthy and sexy.	Psychology of Longevity	2, 3, 4

The Long-Life Personality and Lifestyle Program, continued

Program Goal	Section	Chapter No.
2. Identify sources of stress in your life.	Psychology of Relaxation and Stress Prevention	5, 6
3. Learn step-by-step procedures to relax and insulate yourself from unwanted stress.	Psychology of Relaxation and Stress Prevention	7
4. Learn practical strategies for dealing with the stress of interpersonal relations at home and at work.	Psychology of Relaxation and Stress Prevention	8, 9
5. Develop your own aerobic fitness program that you can follow from now on in order to increase your self-esteem, your vitality and your resistance to disease.	Psychology of Physical Fitness	10
6. Develop your own flexibility program that will stimulate your endocrine system and make you look and feel more youthful.	Psychology of Physical Fitness	11
7. Learn to control your body chemistry to maximize your health and increase stamina and resistance to disease.	Psychology of Controlling Your Body Chemistry	12 to 15
8. Learn the protective properties of specific foods and supplements.	Psychology of Controlling Your Body Chemistry	16

Program Goal	Section	Chapter No.
9. Learn what science says about fasting as a longevity promoter.	Psychology of Controlling Your Body Chemistry	17

NOTES

CHAPTER TWO

The Art, Science And Psychology Of Longevity

How Young Was Methuselah? How Young Are You?

"And Methuselah lived 187 years, and begot Lamech. And Methuselah lived after he begot Lamech 782 years and begot sons and daughters. And all of the days of Methuselah were 969 years."
Genesis 5:25-27.

What's In A Name?

We chose the name *Methuselah Manual* for this book because, according to the Bible, Methuselah lived 969 years. With the help of a little literary conjecture, the story of Methuselah embodies all of the elements that science has established as being part of a long and healthy life.

Because of all the begetting mentioned in the Bible, Methuselah must have had a sizable extended family and many social contacts. No doubt this helped him to develop a strong self-concept. Moreover, he certainly must have believed in something beyond himself to have been written up in the Bible.

Long-Life Factors:
Strong self concept
Extended social contacts
Belief in something beyond self
Mentally and physically fit

Methuselah must have been exceptionally fit, both mentally and physically, in order to handle the wide variety of stresses brought on by the many changes in society over the 969 years that he lived. He probably had a successful career in order to support such a large family.

15

Apparently Methuselah and his wife had such a satisfying sex life that it lasted about 782 years after the birth of their first child, Lamech. We're not saying that Methuselah and his wife lived long only because of their satisfying sex life, but one thing is certain – a satisfying sex life is one of the distinguishing characteristics of the modern-day Methuselahs who have been the object of scientific studies on longevity over the past few decades.

**Satisfying love life.
Good sense of humor.**

Finally, we are willing to bet that he had a good sense of humor and was able to laugh at life and himself. In other words, the quality of Methuselah's life was exceptionally high.

The key factors that promote or prevent you from obtaining vibrant health and long life are illustrated in the lives of real people below. If you are reading this book so that you can spend your time counting the years rather than measuring the quality of the years that will be your life on this earth, perhaps the lessons to be learned from the lives described below will enhance your understanding of how and why some people are eternally young and others are not.

How Old Are These People?

A California man runs 15 miles and then swims and bikes each day. All of this activity takes place before he puts in a full day of physical labor! Weekends are devoted to foot races. He started running when he was 58. He is now in his seventies. Psychologically and biologically, how old is he? Is he younger than you?

A man from western Canada ran in eight marathons in 1983 and participated in one triathalon. According to all reports, he has the body of a 35-year-old man. According to the calendar he is 84. Psychologically and biologically, how old is he? Is he younger than you?

A psychologist runs two miles a day five to six days a week, swims a half-mile two to three times a week, does yoga daily and has two children under 10 years old. He runs his own business, works long hours, flew 100,000 air miles last year and teaches at a major university in Boston. In the last 10 years he has authored over 100 professional publications, including four textbooks. He looks 35 but in reality is 50. Psychologically and biologically, how old is he, really? Is he younger than you?

A New York advertising account executive dropped his successful career to become an author. He was 50 years old. By the time he reached 80, he had written 10 books. Psychologically, how old is this man? Is he younger than you?

A famous software entrepreneur recently dropped dead of a heart attack at age 40. We don't know much about this particular man's lifestyle, but a recent article in a major magazine devoted to computers made a point of underscoring how people in the fast-moving computer business are always bragging about their long, stress-filled hours, their diet of coffee, colas, pizza and tobacco and their lack of exercise, etc. If it is true that the entrepreneur followed the lifestyle described by the computer magazine, then how old do you think he was psychologically and biologically when he died so suddenly at such an early age?

Do you think he was as physically and mentally fit as our 80-year-old marathon runner or our hard-driving psychologist?

More important, really, how old are you?

How Old Are You Psychologically?

The cliché that you are only as old as you feel is absolutely true from a psychological point of view. You are only as old as you think you are, as you behave and as you look and feel. Your personal aging status is not directly related to how old you are in years as much as it is to your physical and mental condition. This includes how productive you are as a worker, parent, friend, lover, spouse, and so on.

Your age is not related to your years. It's related to your physical and mental condition.

Similarly, from a biological point of view, aging is less related to the number of years you have lived than it is to how you function physically.

HOW OLD ARE YOU?
A Psychological Checklist of How Old You Really Are

Directions:
In the situations listed below, indicate how you think you have behaved or would behave in the future. Write down a 1 if you strongly disagree with the statement. Write down a 7 if you strongly agree with the statement. For example, if you think you would never behave in the way the statement suggests, mark down a 1; if you might behave that way about half the time, mark down a 4; if you would definitely behave that way, mark down a 7. Put your score in the score column on the right.

Questions   **Score**

---

1. When I get up in the morning, I look forward to the day ahead.

Strongly Disagree 1-2-3-4-5-6-7 Strongly Agree   ___

2. I feel in control of my life most of the time.

Strongly Disagree 1-2-3-4-5-6-7 Strongly Agree   _5_

3. I am satisfied with the quantity and quality
    of my sex life.

Strongly Disagree 1-2-3-4-5-6-7 Strongly Agree   _5_

4. I would change my job tomorrow if I found
    something more challenging.

Strongly Disagree 1-2-3-4-5-6-7 Strongly Agree   _1_

5. I frequently touch the people I care about.

Strongly Disagree 1-2-3-4-5-6-7 Strongly Agree   _6_

6. I have good friends and an active social life.

Strongly Disagree 1-2-3-4-5-6-7 Strongly Agree   _6_

7. I am good at what I do.

Strongly Disagree 1-2-3-4-5-6-7 Strongly Agree   _6_

8. When I know I am right, I stick to it even
    when other people discourage me.

Strongly Disagree 1-2-3-4-5-6-7 Strongly Agree   _6_

9. I enjoy my job most of the time.

Strongly Disagree 1-2-3-4-5-6-7 Strongly Agree   _6_

10. I enjoy learning and doing new things.

Strongly Disagree 1-2-3-4-5-6-7 Strongly Agree   _7_

A Psychological Checklist of How Old You Really Are

Questions   **Score**

11. I have new career, hobby or personal goals
     for next year.

Strongly Disagree 1-2-3-4-5-6-7 Strongly Agree   _6_

12. I like being alone sometimes to reflect on
     life, to make plans for self-improvement
     or just to think about nothing and relax.

Strongly Disagree 1-2-3-4-5-6-7 Strongly Agree   _7_

13. I feel that the people around my age are
     aging faster than I am.

Strongly Disagree 1-2-3-4-5-6-7 Strongly Agree   _7_

14. I like to have people of all ages involved
     in my life.

Strongly Disagree 1-2-3-4-5-6-7 Strongly Agree   _7_

15. I enjoy physical activities.

Strongly Disagree 1-2-3-4-5-6-7 Strongly Agree   _7_

Scoring the Psychological Well-being Checklist

SCORE
90 - 105

Dale Carnegie, move over! You are a very
positive person and are in charge of your
life. You probably have a supportive social
life and enjoy new challenges. Chances are
you will get a younger-than-your-years
score from your physician on a physiological examination, assuming that your nutritional and exercise programs are as well
balanced as your personality.

76 - 89	You are generally an upbeat person who enjoys life and people. In terms of your physical well-being, you probably look your age but will be "in great shape for your age" if you have taken care of your nutritional and exercise programs.
61 - 75	Life is fair to good. Examine your answers to make sure that your low scores do not cluster into one category, such as work or family or challenges. If they do, then you may want to give that area of your life some thought to determine the cause of your dissatisfaction. The chapters on the psychology of relaxation and stress prevention will be of value to you in determining how you want to change.
46 - 60	Life could be better. There are definitely some areas in your life that could be improved. Whether it is your interpersonal relationships, your career, having challenges in your life or just the way you feel about yourself, you are the best person to determine which area needs your attention. You should stop avoiding the problem and plan a program to address the situation. A physical exam would probably find you in average health for your age with a few physical problems but nothing that couldn't be improved by taking charge of your nutrition and getting more exercise.
0 - 45	The lower your score, the unhappier you are with your life and the more imperative it is that you do something about it. If you feel you cannot cope alone, we suggest a good clinical psychologist or other mental health professional. If you are feeling depressed, start a physical exercise program immediately. Recent research has demonstrated that vigorous physical exercise like running or swimming is very effective for lifting depression. (Make sure you get a physical checkup before beginning any

exercise program. See Chapter 10.) There is a great deal of literature that supports the idea that mental and emotional stress lead to physical illness. We would be willing to bet that a physical exam would find you looking older than your age. If you do not have a serious illness now, research has demonstrated that you stand a good chance of developing one in the next six months if you do not begin to address the causes of stress in your life. This book is an excellent start.

Biologically, How Old Are You?

Medical researchers have come up with a number of indices of aging. Technically, to determine how old you are physically, you will need to have your physician run a series of tests to tell you where you stand on the physical indicators listed below.

1. How much air do you take in in one breath? This indicates your aerobic fitness. Compare this to norms for your chronological age.

Physical indicators of aging.

2. How much blood does your heart pump in its resting state?

3. How well do your kidneys function?

4. Do you look younger or older than most people your age in terms of wrinkles, age spots and skin tone?

5. How quickly do your wounds heal?

6. How fast is your resting pulse?

7. How good are your senses (sight, smell, taste, hearing, touch)?

8. Are you losing calcium from your bones?

9. How good are your reflexes?

There are at least 30 accepted medical tests to measure your degree of physical aging. The ones listed above are probably the most important ones, but they must to be made in a health care environment with appropriate equipment.

For a quick overview of your own degree of aging, you can check yourself out on our "How Old Are You?" self-test. *This is a common-sense test and is over-simplified. It should not be used as a substitute for a good physical before beginning an aerobic program.*

A quick check of how old you are.

HOW OLD ARE YOU?
A Biological Checklist of How Old You Really Are

Questions	Answers	
	Yes	No

---

1. I can do one of the following in 12 minutes:
   a) Run 1.4 miles for men or 1.2 miles for women.
   b) Swim 500 yards for men (10 round trips in an Olympic pool) or 400 yards for women (8 round trips in an Olympic pool.) *

2. I can bend over and touch my toes easily without hurting my back.

3. I can walk up a flight of stairs without puffing.

4. I can walk a mile in about 15 minutes without feeling tired.

A Biological Checklist of How Old You Really Are

Questions	Yes	No
5. I do some kind of physical activity on a regular basis, at least three times a week.	——	——
6. I don't smoke.	——	——
7. I don't drink more than seven drinks a week and not more than three at any one sitting.	——	——
8. I am not more than five pounds over-weight and I get at least seven hours of sleep a night.	——	——
9. I eat very little red meat, fried food or other fatty foods.	——	——
10. I eat lots of fresh fruits, vegetables and whole grains every day.	——	——
11. I avoid white sugar, salt and "junk food".	——	——
12. Most people think I am younger than I am.	——	——
13. I have a lot of energy.	——	——
14. I enjoy a day of vigorous physical activity.	——	——
15. When necessary, I can work long hours without getting moody, over-tired or cranky.	——	——

*Note: According to Kenneth Cooper, M.D., these distances and times put a 40 – 49 year old person in the "good" aerobic category but not in the excellent or superior category. If you are younger or older, you would need to do proportionately more or less to be considered in "good" aerobic shape.

Scoring Yourself

If you can't answer yes to at least 12 of the above questions, you are probably aging physically at a rate that is faster than you would like. Although you can't stop the clock, you *can* slow down the aging process. But only *you* can do it. And that's what this book is about.

What Does Science Say About Why We Age?

The chart below describes some theories of aging. As trained scientists concerned with studying the complex behavior of human beings, we find it difficult to believe that the way to add years to your life can be explained by over-simplified generalizations from research with rats or from nonexperimental research with human beings. However, we believe that we should continue to increase our research efforts on life extension because of the promise it holds for preventive medicine. Ultimately, every new piece of scientific knowledge in the life-extension field can light the way for all of us who want to stay young, healthy and sexy.

Some Theories of Aging

Label	Approach	Proponents
Environmental Theory	Experiments with chicken cells suggested that cells are "immortal" if kept in a waste-free environment. (Note: This theory is no longer considered valid but is included because it was an important theory for many years.)	A. Carrel

Label	Some Theories of Aging, continued Approach	Proponents
Limited Cell Division Theory	Human cells can divide only 50 times, which means that aging is genetically set in the cells. This is not true of cancer cells, which can divide continually and appear to be "immortal."	L. Hayflick
DNA Repair Theory	Genetic material in cells doesn't repair itself fast enough. Rate of repair declines with age.	R. Hart R. Setlow
Free Radicals Theory	Free radicals are chemicals in the cells with an extra charge or electron. They oxidize and destroy cells. Over time the body loses its ability to fight them.	D. Harman
Immunologic Theory	The immune system, the body's system that produces antibodies to fight unwanted invaders, wears out with age. Eventually it turns on itself and attacks the body.	R. Walford
Low Body Temperature Theory	Having a lower body temperature can extend life span. Research with rats has shown that it can work. Some yogis have shown scientists that they can lower body temperature with meditation.	R. Walford Yoga - practitioners
Restricted Food Intake and Fasting Theory	Life span of rats increased up to 40% by restricting calorie intake while providing sound nutrition. Fasting is seen as one method of consistently lowering overall weekly caloric intake. It is also seen by some as a way to purify the system.	P. Airola A. Cott D. Gregory H. Shelton R. Walford Yoga - practitioners
Holistic Theory	Life extension and disease prevention is a complex process which involves lifestyle and the mind and spirit as well as the body.	Russian scientists Yoga - practitioners

The problem with most of these theories is that they try to reduce aging to a simple explanation at the cellular level. We believe that the survival of human beings is a much more complex process than any of us will ever know. You have only to study cases where normal people have performed superhuman feats under psychological pressure or where people have miraculously gained full health from terminal illnesses by using mind control to recognize the current limitations of the behavioral and physical sciences. Actually, of all the biological theories, the only one with well-documented scientific support is the restricted-diet theory. Most of the work has been done with rats, however, and the results have been generalized to human beings.

No one theory completely explains the complex process of human aging.

What Do Centenarians Have in Common?

Besides the knowledge gained from rat, chicken and other animal studies, what else do we know about life extension? As behavioral scientists, we are interested in the comments of people who reached the magic age of 100 and in why they think they made it that far. Over the past 20 years or so, Russian and American scientists have conducted a number of studies of people from societies known for their long-lived people and of actual individuals who have lived to be 100 or more. The chart below summarizes what we believe are the important lessons to be learned from these studies. The encouraging lesson is that many of these people remain physically and mentally fit right up to the end.

What Do Long-Lived People Have In Common?

Variable	Summary	Notes
Diet	Lacto-vegetarian; eat mostly whole grains, vegetables and fruits; dairy is almost always from goat's milk; occasional fish, poultry.	Low fat; high fiber; unrefined carbohydrates; low protein; low calories (about 1800-2000 a day).
Physical Environment	Live in the country in a pollution-free environment. Most live near a large body of water.	Pure water, air, food.
Physical Activity	Do manual labor all day; lots of walking up hills; lots of bending, stretching, lifting.	Deep breathing from physical labor.
Genetics	People with long-lived parents live 3 - 5 years longer than others.	Genetic background is not enough to account for living 30 or 40 extra years.
Tobacco	Smoke home-grown cigar-like tobacco in moderation.	No chemicals in tobacco; do not inhale; do not smoke indoors.
Alcohol	Drink equivalent of about 40 ounces of beer or about a half-bottle of wine per day.	Drinking is spread out over the day and only taken with food, not before meals; home-made brew.

What Do Long-Lived People Have In Common?, continued

Variable	Summary	Notes
Expectations	Expect to live long; are expected to live long by others; expected to contribute to society.	Prefer and seek out the company of active people to keep them stimulated.
Control	Serve as head of household; control the money.	Also have strong religious convictions.
Quality of Lifestyle	Very high quality of life. They enjoy their work!	Not obsessed with time or time pressure.
Social Ties	Lots of social ties; married people out-live unmarried.	People without religious, family or other social ties die sooner than those who have them.

What Does Science Tell Us?

If you want to increase your chances of staying young, healthy and sexy, you are going to have to make some changes in your lifestyle. This next chart is a liberal interpretation and summary of the biological, psychological, and social science research on life extension. The bottom line is that there are ten areas of your life that you must examine and possibly modify in some way if you want to end up with a high quality lifestyle that may add years to your life and which will most certainly add life to your years:

Ten Lifestyle Rules for Staying Young, Healthy and Sexy

1. **LEARN TO EAT RIGHT** — Change your diet to one that gets a large proportion of its calories from whole grains, fresh fruits and vegetables. You may have to cut down considerably on your caloric intake if you are consuming as many calories as most Americans do. You do this automatically and without feeling hungry when you switch to vegetables, fruits and grains.

2. **EXPAND YOUR SOCIAL LIFE** — Develop and maintain a wide circle of people who expect you to live long and to contribute to the family or social unit.

3. **LEARN TO REDUCE STRESS** — Learn to manage the stress in your life, a major cause of cardiovascular deaths and suspected as a cause of other equally debilitating diseases, such as cancer.

4. **MAKE A CONTRIBUTION** — Find an occupation (or a hobby, if your occupation is pretty well solidified) that you feel makes a contribution. It should also be something that can last you well beyond what is now considered the age of retirement.

5. **GET PHYSICALLY FIT** — Institute a physical-fitness program that you can live with the rest of your life. It should provide for aerobic fitness as well as flexibility and deep breathing.

6. **CONTROL YOUR LIFE** — Find a way to stay in control of your life. Surround yourself with people, especially active people, from all age groups.

7. **RELAX** — Learn to relax and take things in stride, and don't get obsessed with time. Laugh at yourself and at life.

8. **STAY IN LOVE** Find a way to maintain a healthy and satisfying sex life.

9. **AVOID JUNK FOOD** Stay away from food with empty calories, preservatives and additives. Learn to read the labels in the food store and make a point of buying foods and water that are free of harmful additives, chemicals and the like.

10. **GET AWAY FROM POLLUTION OR PROTECT YOURSELF FROM IT** If at all possible, move to a pollution-free environment. If this is not possible, find a way to minimize the effects. See the chapters on vitamin supplements and nutrition.

When you add all of the above items to your life, you have the best health insurance anyone can buy. All of these factors have been studied by professionals. Their findings are documented in the scientific journals and reported in popular magazines. Most people have either heard about or read about most of the significant findings on life extension and preventive health care. The question is, "Why aren't more people following these sure-fire directions for staying young, healthy and sexy?" The answer is simple: most people know what they should do, but they don't know how to teach themselves to change. That's what this book is all about.

Most people know what they should do, but they don't know how to teach themselves to change. That's what this book is about.

In order to make these changes, you have to learn to look at things a little differently and to take charge of your life. The next chapter is designed to help you do this so that you can profit from the suggestions presented in the rest of the book.

NOTES

CHAPTER THREE

How Can I Acquire A Long-Life Personality?

Science has established the following characteristics of modern-day Methuselahs: a strong self-concept, physical fitness, competence in their chosen work, a belief in something beyond themselves such as belief in a religion or cause, a sense of humor and, last but not least, a satisfying sex life. In addition, a person with a long-life personality is a person who deals well with change and is able to maintain a lifestyle that is beneficial to his or her mental and physical health.

Let's take a look at the way you handle various situations in your life and find out where you stand.

How Would You Behave?

Directions:

Listed below are some common situations that may occur at work, at home or socially. Think for a minute about how you have behaved in the past in similar situations. Then indicate how you think you have behaved or would behave in the future. Write down a 1 if you strongly disagree with the statement. Write down a 7 if you strongly agree with the statement. For example, if you think you would never behave in the way the statement suggests, mark down a 1; if you might behave that way about half the time, mark it a 4; if you would definitely behave that way, mark it a 7. Put your score in the score column on the right.

Situation   **Score**

1. The next outfit I buy will be the one I like
    best regardless of what the designers are
    offering.

    Strongly Disagree 1-2-3-4-5-6-7 Strongly Agree   _____

2. The next time I'm involved in a disagree-
    ment, I will make every effort to get the
    issues out on the table rather than letting
    things clear up on their own.

    Strongly Disagree 1-2-3-4-5-6-7 Strongly Agree   _____

3. When I work on a difficult project, I try
    to do it myself rather than ask for help.

    Strongly Disagree 1-2-3-4-5-6-7 Strongly Agree   _____

4. The last time I finished a project success-
    fully, I couldn't wait for my co-workers to
    tell me how good it was!

    Strongly Disagree 1-2-3-4-5-6-7 Strongly Agree   _____

5. I prefer TV shows in which the hero works
    on his own.

    Strongly Disagree 1-2-3-4-5-6-7 Strongly Agree   _____

6. When I misunderstand people, it's usually
    their fault because they don't explain
    themselves enough.

    Strongly Disagree 1-2-3-4-5-6-7 Strongly Agree   _____

7. I always do my best work regardless of
    other people's performance.

    Strongly Disagree 1-2-3-4-5-6-7 Strongly Agree   _____

Situation	Score

8. The last time I got a raise I said to myself, "Boy, it's about time; I sure earned this one."

Strongly Disagree 1-2-3-4-5-6-7 Strongly Agree   ————

9. I have always believed that my career success is directly related to my own efforts.

Strongly Disagree 1-2-3-4-5-6-7 Strongly Agree   ————

10. If I hear that someone has made negative comments about me, I don't worry that other people may be thinking the same thing.

Strongly Disagree 1-2-3-4-5-6-7 Strongly Agree   ————

TOTAL SCORE   ————

Scoring:

60 - 70	Strong Sense of Personal Control
50 - 59	Good Sense of Personal Control
40 - 49	Average Sense of Personal Control
Less than 40	Below Desirable Level

If you scored in the 60-70 range, you have a head start on developing a long-life personality! In our opinion, the number one personality factor in stress reduction and life extension is having a sense of control, a *belief* in your own ability to control the factors in your life that make you healthy and happy. Our own research and the research of others verifies this. People who believe that what happens to them is a result of their own actions rather than the result of luck, chance, fate or the whims of powerful others are said to have an internal locus of control. People who believe that the rewards that they get in

The number one personality factor in stress reduction and life extension is the belief in personal control.

life are from luck, chance, fate, powerful others, etc., are said to have an external locus of control.

When we compare these two personality types, there are some incredible differences. People who accept responsibility for their own actions and truly believe that they have to earn what they get are better performers, better workers, more courteous, cooperative, successful, etc. In other words, they are in control. And being in control makes a big difference in the way they handle stress, a major killer!

Research has shown that developing an awareness and understanding of the concept of locus of control is a critical step in learning how to take control of your life and accept the fact that you are ultimately responsible for most of what happens to you. There are a number of studies that have shown that simply finding out about the concept has helped people develop attitudes that are more accepting of personal responsibility.

You are responsible for what happens to you!

There are probably over 3000 published studies on locus of control, ours among them. As part of this research, a number of techniques have been developed for helping people change to the more internal control orientation. The six rules below can serve as guidelines when you feel out of control. One thing we should point out, however, is that you don't always have to have your way in order to have internal control.

Six Rules for Assuming Personal Control of Your Life

1. ACTIVELY ASSUME RESPONSIBILITY   Anytime you catch yourself blaming someone or something else for your choices, sit back and reflect on what you can do to change what happens. How many times have you said, "I can't change what I eat. My wife (or husband or mother) does the shopping and cooking." Or how about, "I'd like to eat like that but I can't cook those kinds of foods. The kids won't eat them." Remember, only those who take responsibility for the outcomes of their behavior have any chance of obtaining and maintaining a long, healthy life. In the chapter on the psychology of interpersonal relations, we discuss how to interact with people in a way that benefits you and them.

2. USE THE LANGUAGE OF RESPONSIBILITY

Take credit for the good and bad. Listen to yourself talk. Are you using phrases like "He made me mad," or "She made me do it"? That kind of talk is the language of a person who does not have an internal orientation. Correct yourself. Say "I was angry with him," or "I did it because I wanted to." Then look at why you chose to be angry with that person or why you chose to do something that you knew would bring you disapproval. Long-life personalities take credit for their own efforts whether the result is success or failure.

3. DISCUSS THE CONCEPT OF TAKING RESPONSIBILITY WITH A PERSON YOU RESPECT

Sit down with someone you really love and who loves you and get them to point out times when you have "copped out." Go over past situations where you let other people or circumstances prevent you from achieving your goals. Ask your loved one and yourself, "Was I more interested in getting approval from others than in attaining my goals? Do I sacrifice what I know is right in order to get the approval of others?"

Of course, everyone needs friends and loved ones. What we are saying here is that giving up what you feel is right because you fear loss of love or loss of approval is not long-life behavior. That kind of behavior leads to feelings of disappointment, anger, resentment and even to serious physical problems. If you find yourself doing this often, try to make up a plan of action to gradually eliminate this type of thinking and behavior. Read the chapter on the psychology of interpersonal skills and try to implement some of the strategies we suggest there.

4. LEARN HOW TO SET GOALS AND DO IT REGULARLY

There is considerable research that shows that goal setting helps people acquire a more internal orientation. Goal setting also helps you perform better. Later on in this chapter we will be talking about goal-setting psychology in more detail.

5. THINK CONNECTIONS!

Understand that almost all of the things that happen to you in life result from choices you have made. Life is a series of stimulus-and-response patterns. We don't continue to respond to stimuli when there are no material or psychological rewards for doing so. You need to examine your response patterns to discover the stimuli that elicit specific behavior patterns from you. Then choose to change those behavior patterns. That's what this book is all about – learning **how** to change.

6. FOCUS ON THE HERE AND NOW

"If only I had..." statements will get you nothing. Instead, ask yourself, "What can I do now to solve a specific problem?" Questions that deal with "now issues" are much more productive and lead to long life.

Scientists and psychologists have tested people's physiological and psychological response to stress. Those who deal best with stress have a characteristic in common with people who live to be 100: while they try to learn from the past and are concerned about the future, basically, they live in the here and now.

"What if..." thinking is equally devastating. This is not to say that planning for the future and working towards future goals is not desirable. There is, however, a very real difference between planning for the future and living for the future. Planning for the future is very important, and we will be discussing it later on in this chapter. Living for the future means that you take no real joy in what is happening today because you are all wrapped up in tomorrow. No one has a guarantee. You could die in an accident five minutes from now. So try to live now. Remember that those who have made it to 100 don't get overly concerned with the future. They may plan for it but they don't worry about it very much. They enjoy life now and have learned to concentrate on being more effective in the present.

How Can I Become More Effective?

The first step is to accept responsibility for your life. Without believing that the things that happen to you are the results of your own actions, your chances of developing a long-life personality are pretty slim. The second step is to learn to practice goal setting, including a perspective that says "I will succeed."

What can goal setting do for me?

Since the late 1930s, psychologists have been researching the relationships between a person's goals and what happens to performance on a variety of tasks and in a variety of situations. Goal setting has proven to be one of the most effective techniques for improving performance.

An Experiment

For example, in one of our experiments, groups of workers who were mentally retarded were randomly assigned to goal-setting conditions or to a control group. By teaching them to set goals, we were able to improve work performance significantly on an assembly task. Before doing goal-setting all of these retarded workers performed well below industry standards. As a result of the goal-setting, some of the retarded workers met and actually exceeded industry standards. The groups who did not set goals continued to perform below standard.

Another important aspect of goal setting is that it highlights the relationship between what you do and what you get. Every time you set a goal, you look for the outcome. This helps to pound home the fact that what you do leads to what you get. Logically, then, goal setting is an excellent technique for helping you develop a more responsible attitude.

Goal setting helps you develop a more responsible attitude.

Goal setting, then, packs a double whammy in terms of what it can do to help you develop a long-life personality and in helping you meet your goals more effectively.

What else can I do to help myself?

You can expect yourself to do well! This probably sounds like a dumb statement, but we want you to think about it. How many times have you set a goal for yourself and immediately heard a little voice inside say, "Hah! You'll never make it!" or "I better not buy that smaller size yet. I don't want to be stuck with a new outfit that's too small." Haven't you just set yourself up to fail?

Think about how many times you say nasty and negative things to yourself. How many times a day do you say things to yourself like, "You dummy! How could you do such a stupid thing?" or "I'm so clumsy!" Or how about, "I'm such a fat slob! I look a mess." etc., etc....

Each of us has a little child inside of us. If you want that child to grow strong and self confident, you must say positive and encouraging things to it. What do you think would happen if you said all those negative things to a real child?

Expect to do well!

An Imaginary Case Study

Imagine that you have a set of identical twins. Because they are identical, everything about them is the same except for the fact that you always speak positively to one and negatively to the other. When twin #1 builds a house with blocks you say, "That's absolutely wonderful. You're such a smart person. I'll bet you can accomplish anything you set out to do." When twin #2 builds the same house you say, "That's a pretty dumb looking house. Why didn't you leave space for a door. How do you expect people to get in and out, stupid? You're not a very good block builder. Why don't you try coloring, but make sure you're not messy like you usually are."

41

Would you really expect the twins to grow up with the same abilities. Of course not. You've beaten poor little twin #2 into the ground. What do you think you are doing to that little kid inside of you when you constantly say negative things to yourself? Give yourself a break! Really listen to the things you say to yourself. Start writing down every negative statement you make to yourself. It will be a shock and should help you become more aware of how much you do it. Examine the negative statements you make, then substitute more positive statements. If you said, "How could I have been so stupid to have made such a careless mistake," try congratulating yourself for catching the error. Say something like, "I'll fix it right away and I'll be more careful next time. I'm usually a very careful person." Try being nice to that poor little kid inside of you. Expect the best and you'll get it.

How Do I Get This Together?

Try the following steps for setting goals and expectation levels by yourself and in cooperation with those around you.

How To Set Effective Goals

---

1. **SET REALISTIC GOALS**

Make sure you set goals you can achieve. While research has shown that people who set goals perform better whether the goal is realistic or not as compared to other people who don't set goals, our experience indicates that it is very helpful to start out setting goals that can be achieved relatively quickly. Don't set yourself up for failure by setting goals that are too general and unachievable in the near future. Goals that are very specific are much easier to accomplish. Let's take a look at some unrealistic goals versus their more specific counterparts.

Which set of goals do you think you could accomplish?

Unrealistic Goals	Realistic Goals
Change my diet and become a vegetarian. (from a person who eats beef 7 days a week)	Eat red meat no more than 5 meals a week including lunch and dinner.
	Buy a vegetarian cookbook by Friday.
	Eat one vegetarian dinner a week.
Start running tomorrow. (from a person who has never done any exercise)	Buy a good pair of running shoes.
	Time myself as I walk one mile as quickly as I can. Based on my time, plan a graduated program.
Stop letting people take advantage of me.	Tell my neighbor I don't mind driving the kids this week if he will drive them next week.
2. **SET GOALS YOU VALUE**	It's self-defeating to set out to accomplish something you don't really value.

Note from Joely

I started running to keep David company and because we couldn't always afford the time to go to the club to swim, which

43

I much prefer as an aerobic activity. However, if I were to be totally honest, I hate running. Since I had asthma as a child, I found running much more difficult than David did. He used to talk about setting goals to get to the next corner, or a certain house, etc. That absolutely did not work for me since I had no desire in the world to get to the next corner or house. I didn't want to be running in the first place, let alone farther along the road. I found that when I tried to set distance goals, I rarely was able to meet them because I didn't really want to run a specific distance. When I gave it some thought, I admitted to myself that I do want to be aerobically fit, and I especially like the effect running has on my thighs. So I began to set goals for calories burned and pulse rate, things that have more value for me. I'm able to accomplish much more with these goals.

3. **WRITE DOWN YOUR GOALS**

We have found that "things to do today" lists are very effective as rewards. Most people get a big kick out of crossing off the completed goals when they finish.

4. **TALK ABOUT YOUR GOALS**

Tell people who will be supportive that you expect to finish this or that by such and such a time. You will be very pleasantly surprised at how much more productive you become when you take charge and tell others you are going to do it!

In a series of classic psychological studies that started in the sixties and continue to the present, it was found that people do better in all kinds of situations when the person in charge *expects* them to do better. This is true of students in a classroom, employees in business, and clients in therapy. Conversely, people will do poorly when the expectations of the supervisor, therapist, teacher or parent are low. Not only can this positive attitude on the part of the person in charge help you do better, but you can also help yourself do better by telling other people your expectation for yourself and getting those around you to set the same expectation.

5. **SET MONTHLY GOALS THEN BREAK THEM DOWN INTO WEEKLY AND DAILY GOALS**

You will perform better and help yourself become more successful at whatever you choose to do. You will also eliminate the anxiety that lots of people have every day when they sit down to go to work. Questions like "What was I supposed to do today?" are immediately answered by a glance at your list of goals and timelines.

Note from Dave and Joely

We are now putting our goals on a computer and have separated the "pages" in the computer file into daily, weekly and long-term goals, as well as personal versus business versus household, etc. Before we got our computer, we used a handy little system called Day-Timers from Allentown, Pennsylvania. Each page contains a goal setting area plus space for appointments, expenses, notes, etc. The system is inexpensive, easy to use, extremely portable, and it comes with a long-range planner so that you can write in goals that go beyond the monthly booklet.

6. **SET PRIORITIES FOR YOUR GOALS**

There are various ways to assign priorities to goals. You can rank order them (1st, 2nd, 3rd, etc.) or assign letters to them

45

(A = Top, B = Next, C = Lowest, and add numbers – A1, A2, A3, etc.). Deal first with "A" priorities. However, remember that A-priority goals can become C-priority goals and vice versa over time.

7. **WORK ON ONLY ONE GOAL AT A TIME**

During your daily activities, work on a top-priority goal until you can go no farther that day. Then start the next-highest-priority goal, and so on. Sequencing and prioritizing are very important. Only you can do it. Remember, you are in charge of your life. If you assign a priority sequence to a goal and want to change it after some experience, then change it! No harm done. The important thing is to think about what you want to do, to believe that you can make it happen and to do it now!

8. **EXPECT TO FALL OFF THE WAGON OCCASIONALLY**

Nobody's perfect. Even with the best of intentions and all the motivation in the world, you will probably slip off the straight and narrow path you have set for yourself. So what! Pick yourself up, dust yourself off, and continue where you left off. Notice we didn't say that you should start all over again. You don't have to start all over again. You already started. Just because you stopped for a little while doesn't take away that fact. All you have to do is continue. Don't forget to congratulate yourself for picking yourself up and having the courage and perseverance to start again. You deserve it.

This Sounds Wonderful, But...?

You're thinking at this point that it all sounds wonderful, except that every time you've tried to get rid of a bad habit or change the way you react to certain things or situations, you end up failing and feeling miserable. Join the group. You are absolutely normal! Everyone who tries to implement change in his or her life finds resistance. The source of the resistance is within and is influenced by those around us. The next chapter will show you how to deal more effectively with your own natural tendency to resist change.

NOTES

_____

_____

_____

_____

_____

_____

_____

_____

_____

_____

_____

_____

_____

_____

_____

_____

_____

_____

_____

NOTES

CHAPTER FOUR

Dealing With Your Natural Tendency To Resist Change

More on Goals and Behavior Control

Without training, most people are not able to make permanent changes in their lifestyle, especially when it involves teaching themselves to exercise regularly, eat different foods and handle the people in their lives differently. However, by learning the simple rules of behavior control, most people can make the necessary changes that will help them develop a long-life personality and stay young, healthy and sexy.

What Do I Need to Know in Order to Help Myself?

This question brings to mind the joke about how many therapists it takes to change a light bulb. The answer: Only one...but the light bulb really has to want to change. If down deep you really don't want to develop a long-life personality, no amount of technology from the social or physical sciences is going to work for you.

Do you really want to change?

You also need to remember that the bad habits you have are the result of learnings that took place some time ago. It takes time to develop a different response pattern. It takes conscious thought to break a negative response pattern. You can do this only if you are truly motivated to make the change.

Assuming that you have decided to take charge of your life, the trick is to find the best method to substitute new learning and good habits for old learning and bad habits.

Substitute good habits for old, bad habits.

How Can I Change My Habits to Stay Young, Healthy and Sexy?

The techniques of self behavior modification below are based on several decades of research geared to helping people learn to behave in ways that will benefit them. When you try one of these techniques, give yourself enough time to measure your progress. If it doesn't seem to work after you have given yourself enough time, don't get discouraged. Try combining this technique with another one or start a new approach altogether.

Eleven Techniques For Changing Your Behavior

1. **SET A VERY SPECIFIC LONG-TERM GOAL THAT CAN BE MEASURED**

Before you can change a behavior, you have to have an outcome that you can measure to see if you have accomplished your goal. The key is to be very specific about what your goal is. Some examples of vague goals and measurable goals are listed below.

Example of a poorly stated goal:
I will improve my eating habits.

Example of a measurable goal:
At the end of three months from today I will no longer eat white sugar or things made with white sugar.

Example of a poorly stated goal:
I am going to do some aerobic exercise every day.

Example of a measurable goal:
At the end of four months, I will be jogging two miles per day a minimum of four days a week.

As you can see from the examples above, measurable goals are very specific. You or anyone else can check on them quite simply. When long-term measurable goals are combined with short-term measurable goals, it creates a very powerful change technique.

2. **BREAK YOUR LONG-TERM GOAL INTO SPECIFIC SHORT-TERM GOALS**

It is easier to get to the long-term goals if you can make up subsidiary short-term goals. These short-term goals serve as stepping stones or check-points that you can monitor on the way to achieving your final goal. Let's say that you want to eliminate sugar from your diet. You might set up a series of short-term goals that look like this:

1. The first week, I will remove all products from my kitchen that contain sugar or sucrose and substitute products that do not contain sugar. (You can buy sugarless ketchup in any health food store that tastes as good as sugared ketchup. Even the kids won't know the difference.)

2. The second week, I will no longer put white sugar in my coffee except for the first cup in the morning.

3. The third week and thereafter, I will drink my coffee without white sugar.

The idea is to take the time to develop a series of short-term achievable successes that eventually lead to the elimination of the unwanted habit and the substitution of a good one.

3. **REWARD YOURSELF** In psychology, the concept of rewarding yourself or being rewarded by others for achieving a desired behavior is called positive reinforcement. Of all the techniques for changing behavior, this is probably the most powerful one. It works best when the reward is given immediately after you have achieved your short-term goal. For example, you could treat yourself and go out after dinner and buy a new color of nail polish if you don't eat dessert tonight.

The rewards don't have to be big deals. They could include buying a new paperback to read, or treating yourself to a candlelit bubblebath.

Note from Joely

I'm allergic to any kind of physical exercise. As a child I paid special attention to my mother's statement that ladies don't sweat, they glisten, and have studiously avoided all activities that produced anything faintly resembling sweat. However, I finally admitted that if I wanted to stay young, healthy and sexy I would have to get involved in physical activity. I reward myself for going to the health club by taking a nice long steam bath. It gives me something to look forward to while I run or swim.

Note from Dave

One of the hardest things I do is to write against a tight deadline. As consulting psychologists and authors, Joely and I frequently are caught in situations where something must be produced "overnight" for a business client. One of my favorite behavior-modification tricks is to set up some low-priority goals for the week. These goals have nothing to do with getting the report or book chapter done by the end of the week. Instead, they are little things I like to do around the house, like hanging the new picture in my daughter's room, playing with some new software on my computer, etc. These goals then become my rewards for getting to a certain spot in a chapter or report. For example, right now my reward for finishing this chapter is to take the time tomorrow to make a scratching pad for our new kitten!

4. **MAKE SURE THE REWARD CONFLICTS WITH THE BAD HABIT**

Your reward for not eating dessert should involve something that has nothing to do with food. Ideally the reward would involve some sort of activity such as playing tennis, or going for a walk with your spouse or going to the roller skating rink with the kids. When Joely first started running, she rewarded herself by making up a body measurement chart and recording measurements on a weekly basis. Every sixteenth of an inch lost was a reward in itself.

5.	**CHANGE THE SCENE**	This technique is very effective in getting rid of a bad eating, drinking or smoking habit. Keep a record of when and where you are most likely to eat that favorite dessert or have that drink. Tell yourself that from now on you can only have dessert or the drink in a place that is inconvenient. Stick to it! After a while you may forgo the dessert or the drink because it's just too much trouble to go to the place you are now allowing yourself to eat or drink this prohibited item.
6.	**CHALLENGE YOURSELF**	Make the whole thing a challenge. Research shows that those who view change as an opportunity or challenge are more likely to be resistant to mental and physical illness brought on by stress!
7.	**FIND A HERO OR HEROINE**	There is an enormous body of research that shows that people can improve their performance and learning by watching other people perform. The catch is that this person must be someone who is significant in your life. Find yourself a person or group of people who have the good habits that you want to acquire and follow their lead. You'd be surprised how much this can speed up your program and give you added zeal!
8.	**GET YOUR LOVED ONES INVOLVED**	Staying motivated is a key to successful habit change. Try to get someone close to you to agree to do it with you and to help you monitor your own behavior.

Note from Joely

Remember, your goal is to make a permanent change. The worst thing you can do to yourself is to lose fifty pounds in a short space of time and then put it back on in about the same space of time. This is bad for your health and for your self esteem. If your loved one will go along with you in a program, it will be much easier for you. Who knows, you may help your loved one more than you think by helping yourself. If you think there will be any resistance, you need to be persuasive and set an example. For heaven's sake, don't nag. That's the kiss of death to cooperation. Although I initiated many of the nutritional changes in our lives, I'll be the first to admit that it was David's influence that got me into the aerobic program. He kept saying things like, "I really like it when you run with me. It makes me feel good." That was about the only thing that made it worthwhile in the beginning. See! Even psychologists go for that positive reinforcement stuff!

9. **EVALUATE AND REEVALUATE**

The idea here is to keep talking to yourself (and your loved one) about the situation and monitor it continuously. Try to come up with new ways to handle social situations where you find it difficult to keep to the goal. For example, if you end up eating food with sugar in it because you go bowling on Thursday nights, you can change the situation. One way would be to bring along a sugar-free snack to substitute for the "junk food" your friends eat. If you want to cut down on the liquor that you drink when you are out, order sparkling water and lime. It gives you something to hold and something bubbly to drink. Or try ordering one of the nonalcoholic beers that are becoming more and more popular. Our favorite is a brand called Moussy. It tastes like beer and has a lot fewer calories.

10. **SEE YOURSELF AS A WINNER** When you are in a relaxed state, do a controlled daydream: visualize yourself meeting your goal. Actually see yourself accomplishing the goal and telling people about it. See people talking to you about how you did it and congratulating you on your success. **It's a very powerful technique.** There are step-by-step directions in Chapter 7.

11. **POST A LIST** Make up a list of the goals you have set for yourself. If you can, get the list typed so it's more official. List the habit changes, target dates for short- and long-term goals and the rewards. Post it where you will see it every day. Make additional copies. Tape one to the bathroom mirror, put one on your wall at work and carry one in your briefcase.

Sample Goals And Rewards For Aerobics

Goals	Rewards

Long-Term Goal

To be running 2 miles in 20 minutes within six months

Buy myself a new gortex running suit (or something else I've wanted, like a special tool or a facial).

Short-Term Goals – This Week

Buy running shoes.

Use my car odometer to set up a two-mile course near home.

Goals	Rewards
Check out health clubs.	For each day that I meet the goal I can watch a rental movie of my choice.
See how quickly I can walk 2 miles.	
Walk 2 miles at least three times this week.	

Next Week

Goals	Rewards
Start a running program as outlined in Chapter 11.	
Walk/run four times this week.	Invite Jack and Sheila over for a game of Trivial Pursuit.

Sample Goals And Rewards For Diet Changes

Goals	Rewards

Long-Term Goal

Goals	Rewards
Within three months only 30% of my calories will come from fat.	Instead of taking in my clothes myself, I'll bring them to a seamstress.

Short-Term Goal - This Week

Goals	Rewards
Buy a low-fat cookbook.	
Try three low-fat recipes this week.	
Use sugar-free jam on my toast instead of butter.	Treat myself to a new kind of bread from the health food store.

CHAPTER FOUR WORKSHEET

LONG-LIFE PERSONALITY GOALS AND REWARDS

Long Term Goal(s)   Rewards

_____

_____

_____

_____

Short Term Goals   Rewards

_____

_____

_____

_____

_____

_____

_____

_____

_____

_____

_____

_____

Reminder Notes:

_____

_____

_____

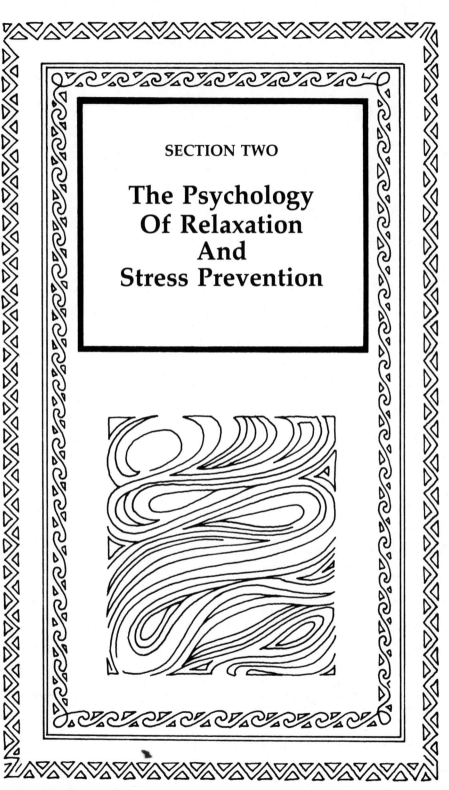

SECTION TWO

The Psychology
Of Relaxation
And
Stress Prevention

The Psychology Of Personal Stress

Americans take aspirin literally by the millions of tons each year.

Over half of the deaths in this country are from heart attacks.

The most widely prescribed drugs are tranquilizers.

If you sit in a steam room with a group of average American males, undoubtedly you'll hear stories of a recent heart attack, an ulcer kicking up or a divorce in the making.

All of these conditions can be caused or aggravated by stress. This section will teach you skills that will help you develop your own long-life personality. In particular, you'll learn how to relax in a way that will have a positive impact on your body's ability to deal with stress. You'll also begin to learn how to use these techniques to help you gain a sense of personal control.

What Is Stress Anyway?

Do you remember that close call you had in the car when some nut almost ran you off the road in the middle of a storm? Remember how your heart started pounding, how you could hardly get enough air in your lungs, how your palms got all sweaty and how you almost threw up afterward? Boy, were you scared! Well, that's stress!

Do you remember the last time you had an important meeting at 9 a.m. and got stuck in the expressway traffic? That's also stress.

How about the time you were having the family reunion at your house? Even though you were glad to be doing it and excited about seeing everyone, organizing it was stressful.

Is Stress Always Bad?

Your response to stress can be (1) neutral, (2) bad for you or (3) good for you.

Stress is not always bad for you.

Simple things like walking or breathing put stress on specific muscles. This kind of stress is considered neutral since it helps you adapt to your everyday environment.

Stress can be bad for you when your reaction leads to negative changes in your body chemistry or mental state. These changes can lead to illness or disease. For example, the stress of a poor diet can lead to a heart attack; the stress of too much worry could lead to an ulcer, etc.

Stress can be good for you when it improves your performance or functioning. Research has shown that moderate stress improves performance. Think about it. If there is so little stress surrounding a specific project that you feel absolutely no time pressure, no pressure to do a good job, no need to extend yourself even the slightest, in all likelihood you will not perform at your very best. On the other hand, moderate stress gives you enough of an adrenaline boost to enhance your performance without overloading your system. So don't think of stress as all bad.

Moderate stress improves performance.

What Causes Stress?

The causes of stress fall into three broad categories:

1. **PHYSICAL**

Physical causes of stress are in the environment. They include contaminated food, polluted air and water, radiation, noise, extremes of temperature, injuries, etc. In most cases, you have the option to avoid or remediate many of these if you want to take charge of your life and are willing to expend the energy to do so.

2. **SOCIAL**

Social causes of stress come from everyday living. Some of them are unavoidable and are part of being human, such as the death of a loved one, the loss of a job or a divorce. For a social cause of stress to be harmful to you, it doesn't have to be valued as negative. Happy stressful events, such as a marriage, a promotion, a vacation, or the birth of a baby can cause psychological and physiological responses that are indistinguishable from responses caused by negative events. Your body does not distinguish between negatively loaded events and positively loaded events in its response.

3. **PSYCHOLOGICAL**   Your own feelings are the psychological causes of stress. They include such feelings as worry, anger, hate, love, fear, inferiority, anxiety and frustration.

Ten Signs of Stress

Whether it is the danger of some wild animal attacking you in the forest or your boss firing you, your body reacts basically the same way to all stressful events. This response to stress is called the "fight or flight" response. It can cause you to have all or some of the following symptoms.

1. **AN INCREASED HEART RATE**   Remember how your heart pounded when you asked someone out socially for the first time?

2. **TREMENDOUS CHANGES IN BREATHING RATE**   Love songs that say "she takes my breath away" are describing this stress response.

3. **SWEATY PALMS, PERSPIRATION**   The next time you go for an interview, dry your hands just before you shake hands with the interviewer. He or she is trained to look for signs of nervousness!

4. **SHIVERING, TREMBLING**   If you are cold or trembling all the time without any physical cause, you are probably experiencing a stress response.

5. **SURGING FEELINGS**   Remember your feelings of anger and fear when you were almost in an automobile accident?

6. **TENSE MUSCLES**   Do you have a knot in the back of your neck or between your shoulder blades? Are your shoulders constantly raised?

7.	**CHANGES IN HOW YOU PERCEIVE THINGS**	You can have blurred vision as a result of stress, or it can affect your psychological perception of things. For example, you might even see things happening more slowly than they really are.
8.	**INCREASED OR DECREASED ABILITY TO CONCENTRATE**	Increased ability to concentrate or pay attention. If you have ever gone fishing, you know the feeling when the fish hits your line! Your whole being is focused on that one event! On the negative side, stress can prevent you from being able to concentrate at all.
9.	**TERRIBLE THINGS IN YOUR TUMMY**	Your gastrointestinal tract basically shuts down. You may get nausea or other symptoms.
10.	**DRY MOUTH OR TONGUE**	Ever notice how many public speakers keep a glass of water nearby?

All of these reactions to stress are there to help you survive. They evolved over millions of years, giving you the ability either to run away from danger or to stay and fight for your life. The problem with these reactions comes when you have them all the time. Your body can recover from acute stress only so many times without making you sick.

The chart below summarizes the hard facts about stress.

 Five Facts About Stress

1.	**STRESS IS IMPARTIAL**	The source of your stress does not have to be valued as negative to have negative effects on your body. Good stress can have just as negative an effect on you as bad stress.

2.	**STRESS IS CUMULATIVE**	Stress can build up inside you and then come out as either mental or physical "disease" or both. Since stress is impartial, a series of good things happening to you can have the same cumulative effect as a series of negative events.
3.	**STRESS AFFECTS THE MUSCLES**	Stress can cause muscle cramps in your legs, arms and other areas of your body. This can throw your body out of balance. Poor posture can lead to some serious physical problems. Also, when your muscles are tense, they are more easily injured.
4.	**STRESS AFFECTS THE MIND**	Stress can cause you to have all kinds of mental problems. A common problem is lying in bed awake all night. During this time you relive in living color all of the things that happened to you that day, or you spend the whole night planning out what you will do the next day.
5.	**STRESS AFFECTS THE GUT**	Stress can hit you hard in your gut. Heartburn, gas, diarrhea, constipation, etc., are common reactions to a stress overload. If these reactions become chronic, they can lead to more serious diseases.

Stress and What You Think About

There are a number of research studies that suggest that what people think about and what they feel about themselves directly affects their health. Research indicates that when you hold a personally harmful set of beliefs like "No one ever appreciates me," in time it may lead to disease. Of course, the opposite is also true. If you hold a positive set of beliefs about yourself and your life, you are more likely to stay healthy. Take a look at the chart on the next page and decide if you have any of these thoughts and feelings.

Do You Feel This Way?

1. I'm always being nagged at.   __X__ Yes   _____ No

2. I stick in there even if I hate it.   __X__ Yes   _____ No

3. I want the job done now!   __X__ Yes   _____ No

4. My parents neglected me.   __X__ Yes   _____ No

5. I always get what I want.   _____ Yes   __X__ No

6. I always control my anger.   _____ Yes   __X__ No

7. Everybody mistreats me.   __X__ Yes   _____ No

8. I like to achieve my goals and then relax.   __X__ Yes   _____ No

9. I never get what I deserve, but I will get even.   _____ Yes   __X__ No

10. I'm afraid I'll get injured.   __X__ Yes   _____ No

11. I just have too much responsibility.   __X__ Yes   _____ No

12. I feel like I can't move or do anything, like I'm chained to life.   __X__ Yes   _____ No

Scoring

Beside each question number below is a brief description of what research has shown about the relationship between symptoms or diseases and feelings, beliefs and attitudes. Note that these are studies of people "on the average." Therefore, it doesn't mean that you'll get or have the symptom if you hold a specific belief. What it means is that you have a higher risk of getting that symptom or disease.

Question	Response
1.	If you answered yes, then you run a higher risk of skin problems, like acne or psoriasis.
2.	If you answered yes, then you may may be suffering from constipation.
3.	If you answered yes, you could have problems with diarrhea.
4.	A yes answer means a higher risk of asthma.
5.	People who answered yes to this one run the risk of frequent heartburn.
6.	A yes answer means you could have or get a hernia.
7.	Hives are associated with a yes answer.
8.	People who can't relax until they have achieved their goals frequently suffer from migraine headaches.
9.	A yes answer indicates the liklihood of getting an ulcer.
10.	A yes answer indicates a higher risk of high blood pressure.
11.	You may suffer from fluid buildup in your body if you answered yes to this question.
12.	People who feel restricted often suffer from rheumatoid arthritis.

How about Stress and My Personality?

There are many theories about the relationship between personality types and illnesses and some correlational research evidence to support these theories. Take a look and see if you find yourself described in any one of the eight scenarios in the chart below.

Is This Your Personality?

---

1. I'm hardworking and conscientious, but I'm not that happy inside.   ___X___ Yes   _____ No

2. You wouldn't believe how nice I keep my things. Everything is in order and neat. I'm always on time and like everything to be perfect. However, I'm easily frustrated.   _____ Yes   ___X___ No

3. Because I'm so neat, people think of me as prim. But I'm nice to be around because I'm mild mannered and conscientious. I hold back my anger.   _____ Yes   ___X___ No

4. I run in "lowgear" and hold back my emotions. I'm depressed a lot.   ___X___ Yes   _____ No

5. I'm very aggressive and I'm angry a lot. I don't really like my situation or most people. I also tend to punish myself.   _____ Yes   ___X___ No

6. I'm a very well-mannered person and very conscientious. I tend to be over-dependent on others. I'm a mild sort of person.   ___X___ Yes   _____ No

7. I'm an achiever and very competitive. I'm extremely compulsive about getting my goals accomplished. People think of me as "hard driving." I never let the fact that I'm tired get in the way of work.   _____ Yes   ___X___ No

8. I know that I am in control of my   ✓ Yes _____ No
    life. While I like to be with other
    people and they like to be with me, I
    make my own decisions and act
    accordingly. I am committed to my
    career and my loved ones and enjoy
    new challenges. Even though I love
    my work, I keep it in perspective.
    I'm able to find time to spend with my
    family. I work out almost every day,
    and I spend time alone meditating on
    my life.

Scoring

Each question should be examined individually. Remember, people are not exactly alike and your personality may not be accurately described by any one of the scenarios listed above. However, on the average, research has shown that people who behave as described above are more likely to contract a specific disease or to maintain a certain physical condition.

Question		Response
1.	Yes	Hardworking but unhappy people usually suffer from depression.
2.	No	A yes answer indicates the risk of getting rheumatoid arthritis.
3.	No	A personality like this one may give you an ulcer.
4.	Yes	People who hold back their emotions are more likely than others to contract cancer.
5.	No	A yes answer suggests that you may be accident-prone.
6.	Yes	If you are like this you may already suffer from ulcerative colitis.

Question	Response
7. No	Hard driving people who don't know when or how to relax often end up as victims of heart attacks.
8. yes	If you are like this, you probably have much of the stress in your life under control. If fact, you have what we call a long-life personality.

CHAPTER FIVE NOTES

_____
_____
_____
_____
_____
_____
_____
_____
_____
_____
_____
_____
_____
_____
_____
_____
_____
_____
_____
_____
_____
_____
_____
_____

NOTES

CHAPTER SIX

Determining The Sources Of Stress In Your Life

Stress that is not handled properly can affect you in many ways. It can impair your ability to function mentally at home and at work. You can experience a variety of physical symptoms that can range from headaches to gastro-intestinal upsets. Everyone experiences the negative effects of stress at various points in their lives. The danger lies in chronic stress overload. When your body is constantly in the fight or flight mode, you are bound to blow a fuse at your body's weakest point. For some people the end result is a serious mental or physical illness.

When you are constantly under stress, you are bound to blow a fuse at your body's weakest point.

The multi-part survey in this chapter is designed to help you determine:

1. Your general level of stress.

2. Your level of stress at work.

3. Your physical symptoms of stress.

4. Your level of stress in interpersonal situations.

Take a look at the checklists that follow to see how stressed you are.

HOW STRESSED ARE YOU?

Directions:

Indicate how often your feelings agree with the statements below. Scoring for each item is based on the following scale:

1 = Never feel that way
2 = Seldom feel that way
3 = Sometimes feel that way
4 = Frequently feel that way
5 = Always feel that way

HOW STRESSED ARE YOU?
General Feelings

Is This You?   **How Often?**

1. I worry a lot.   Never 1-2-3-4-5 Always

2. I feel unhappy.   Never 1-2-3-4-5 Always

3. All kinds of worrisome thoughts
   run through my mind.   Never 1-2-3-4-5 Always

4. I imagine scary things.   Never 1-2-3-4-5 Always

5. There are times when I feel like
   crying for no reason.   Never 1-2-3-4-5 Always

6. There are times when I can't react to
   anything; I'm frozen in time and space.   Never 1-2-3-4-5 Always

7. Life seems so unreal.   Never 1-2-3-4-5 Always

8. I don't know what's the matter with
   me. I'm so irritable all the time.   Never 1-2-3-4-5 Always

General Feelings

Is This You?	How Often?

9. I have lost my ability just to sit
    around and do nothing. Never 1-2-3-4-5 Always

10. I feel like I'm living inside a pressure
    cooker and am about to explode. Never 1-2-3-4-5 Always

11. I've finally realized that people just
    have to pick on me all the time. Never 1-2-3-4-5 Always

12. Lately I'm bored with my life, my job,
    my friends and even my loved ones. Never 1-2-3-4-5 Always

13. Deep inside, I'm dissatisfied and I
    don't know why. Never 1-2-3-4-5 Always

14. I forget things. Never 1-2-3-4-5 Always

Total Score = _____ 46

HOW STRESSED ARE YOU?

Work Performance

Is This You?	How Often?

1. I have trouble concentrating on my
    work. Never 1-2-3-4-5 Always

2. It takes me forever to make decisions. Never 1-2-3-4-5 Always

3. I can't seem to stick to a job. Never 1-2-3-4-5 Always

4. I pace around all the time at work. Never 1-2-3-4-5 Always

5. From the time I get there until I leave,
    I'm plain fidgety. Never 1-2-3-4-5 Always

6. I overreact to things at work. Never 1-2-3-4-5 Always

Work Performance

Is This You?	How Often?
7. I let minor things get to me.	Never 1-2-3-4-5 Always
8. I procrastinate.	Never 1-2-3-4-5 Always
9. I can't seem to get organized.	Never 1-2-3-4-5 Always
10. I don't seem to judge people right.	Never 1-2-3-4-5 Always
11. I'm unclear about my role here.	Never 1-2-3-4-5 Always
12. I work long hours and bring work home.	Never 1-2-3-4-5 Always
13. I do a lot of paper shuffling.	Never 1-2-3-4-5 Always
14. I don't trust anyone at work.	Never 1-2-3-4-5 Always

Total Score = _____

HOW STRESSED ARE YOU?
Physical Symptoms

Is This You?	How Often?
1. My heart races or pounds.	Never 1-2-3-4-5 Always
2. I get chest pains, but my heart is fine.	Never 1-2-3-4-5 Always
3. I have trouble catching my breath.	Never 1-2-3-4-5 Always
4. I get diarrhea.	Never 1-2-3-4-5 Always
5. I have headaches.	Never 1-2-3-4-5 Always
6. I have to urinate frequently.	Never 1-2-3-4-5 Always
7. I get dizzy for no reason.	Never 1-2-3-4-5 Always

HOW STRESSED ARE YOU?, continued
Physical Symptoms

Is This You?	How Often?

8. I have no appetite.

Never 1-2-3-4-5 Always *(1 circled)*

9. I spend my nights awake, or it takes forever to fall asleep.

Never 1-2-3-4-5 Always *(2 circled)*

10. I'm tired.

Never 1-2-3-4-5 Always *(4 circled)*

11. My throat and/or mouth is often dry.

Never 1-2-3-4-5 Always *(3 circled)*

12. I sigh a lot.

Never 1-2-3-4-5 Always *(2 circled)*

13. My stomach is tense.

Never 1-2-3-4-5 Always *(3 circled)*

14. I have no energy.

Never 1-2-3-4-5 Always *(4 circled)*

15. I'm chilly.

Never 1-2-3-4-5 Always *(1 circled)*

16. I actually throw up for no reason.

Never 1-2-3-4-5 Always *(1 circled)*

17. My neck (or shoulders, eyes, chest, lower back, throat, hands) is sore, stiff or painful.

Never 1-2-3-4-5 Always *(5 circled)*

18. Lately I seem to have one bug or cold after another.

Never 1-2-3-4-5 Always *(2 circled)*

19. I grind my teeth in my sleep.

Never 1-2-3-4-5 Always *(2 circled)*

20. In the afternoon I run out of steam.

Never 1-2-3-4-5 Always *(3 circled)*

21. My posture is terrible.

Never 1-2-3-4-5 Always *(3 circled)*

Total Score = ___58___

HOW STRESSED ARE YOU?
Interpersonal Relations

Is This You?   **How Often?**

1. I startle easily when people come up
    on me.   Never 1-2-3-4-5 Always

2. I cry over little things.   Never 1-2-3-4-5 Always

3. I blush easily around people.   Never 1-2-3-4-5 Always

4. Around people, I can't speak correctly.   Never 1-2-3-4-5 Always

5. When someone gets me upset, I feel
    like I'm going faint.   Never 1-2-3-4-5 Always

6. I can't stand to be around a particular
    person (or group).   Never 1-2-3-4-5 Always

7. I can't stand to be around people
    when they are emotional!   Never 1-2-3-4-5 Always

8. I can't tell anyone how I feel.   Never 1-2-3-4-5 Always

9. I don't feel anything.   Never 1-2-3-4-5 Always

10. I can't laugh at myself.   Never 1-2-3-4-5 Always

11. Down deep, I'm not happy with my
    sex life.   Never 1-2-3-4-5 Always

12. I don't trust anybody.   Never 1-2-3-4-5 Always

Total Score = 24

78

HOW STRESSED ARE YOU? SCORING SHEET

Category	No. Items	Total Score (Add Up All Items)	Average Score (Divide Total Score by Number of Items)
General Feelings	14	46	
Work Performance	14		
Physical Symptoms	21	58	
Interpersonal Relations	12	24	
ALL SCALES *	61	128	2.

* To compute overall average score, add up your total scores for each scale and divide by 61.

How To Interpret Your Scores On Individual Sections

General Feelings

14 – 28 = Low Stress
29 – 42 = Moderate Stress
42 – 56 = High Stress
57 – 70 = Very High Stress

Work Performance

14 – 28 = Low Stress
29 – 42 = Moderate Stress
42 – 56 = High Stress
57 – 70 = Very High Stress

Physical Symptoms

21 – 42 = Low Stress
43 – 63 = Moderate Stress ✓
64 – 84 = High Stress
85 – 105 = Very High Stress

Interpersonal Problems

12 – 24 = Low Stress ✓
25 – 36 = Moderate Stress
37 – 48 = High Stress
49 – 60 = Very High Stress

Total average scores below 3 are okay, but you should strive to get yourself into the 2's. Of course, there will be periods in your life when your score will climb temporarily because you run into stressful situations that are out of your control. In many cases you can learn new ways to deal with these stressful events so that the next time you are faced with one, you will react in a more relaxed fashion.

Be careful that you don't overreact and create a stressful event out of scoring and interpreting these scales. At one time or another, all of us are bound to have some of the symptoms listed in the four categories above. However, every one of the items on these checklists is a sign of stress if you scored yourself 4 or higher. You will probably want to look at those items to see where you can begin to make changes. If you can't think of any specific thing you can do to change the item, look at the list again after you have finished this book.

Note from Dave and Joely

Sometimes the source of the stress is easily explained and right in front of your nose. For example, one of our clients confided to us that he was experiencing terrible stress symptoms. When we questioned him more closely, he admitted to feeling out of breath on occasion, to having blurred vision once in a while, to having frequent indigestion, to being unable to sleep, and generally, to feeling terribly anxious. He was very involved with overseeing a major reorganization of his department. He was a man who had directed several similar automation projects and attributed his gastrointestinal problems to the real work stress he was undergoing. We observed his behavior over a period of several days and noted that he drank about 10 cups of coffee a day without even thinking. We bought him a hot water heater and a variety of herbal tea bags. The symptoms cleared up immediately and only came back when he lapsed into his old coffee-drinking habit!

Okay, So I'm Under Stress. What Can I Do About It?

Since the only way to fully eliminate stress is to die, we must all learn to live with and control the stress in our lives. You can eliminate stress or reduce its effects by:

1. Keeping yourself physically fit.
    See Section Three.

2. Improving your nutrition.
    See Section Four.

3. Learning to relax and to interact more effectively with people. Chapters 7, 8 and 9 focus on these areas.

CHAPTER SIX NOTES

CHAPTER SEVEN

The Psychology Of Personal Relaxation

According to the dictionary, rest is the act of ceasing from work or activity. Relaxation, however, has a more profound meaning. One meaning of relaxation is the lengthening of inactive muscles. As we discuss in the chapter on flexibility, lengthening the muscle fibers releases muscle tension and allows for improved blood and oxygen flow throughout your entire body. A second definition of relaxation actually comes out of the physical sciences but can be said to describe the psychological effects of a relaxation program. This definition talks about relaxation as being the return of a system to equilibrium. This is exactly what a relaxation program will do for you. It will bring your entire system back to equilibrium.

Relaxation has a more profound meaning than rest.

A Rose By Any Other Name...

Relaxation programs have been studied under a variety of names: the relaxation response, self-hypnosis, focused concentration, transcendental meditation, active meditation, passive meditation, etc. To the uninitiated, they are very similar, and to be sure, the results obtained from any of these methods are essentially the same. Throughout this chapter, we'll refer to our relaxation program simply as meditation.

There has been a great deal of interest in the effects of meditation on psychological and physical well-being. These effects have been studied using the latest scientific methods. The list below summarizes the findings.

Scientifically Established Benefits of Meditation

Physical benefits of meditation.

* Lower cholesterol
* Slower heart rate
* Decreased chances of heart attack
* Decreased oxygen consumption
* Reduced blood pressure
* Decreased breathing rate
* Increased relief from asthma
* Increased relief from bronchitis
* Increased saliva, which aids digestion
* Decreased incidence of irregular heartbeats
* Increased muscle relaxation
* Increased electrical resistance of skin, which means less anxiety

---

Implementing The 3% Formula for Meditation

You can have all of the benefits of meditation by spending only 20 minutes a day six days a week. How many mornings do you lay in bed dreading to get up? You can use that time to meditate and get out of bed feeling immeasurably better than if you just laid there wishing time would stand still. How many nights do you sit down to watch a television program in order to relax and get up feeling more tired than when you sat down? For a 20 minute investment of your time in the morning or evening you can feel calmer, more refreshed, and more excited about dealing with life. It's one of the best investments you can make.

Note from Dave

The first time I tried meditation the effects were immediate. At that time, I was a young, uptight corporate marketing manager, the typical Type A personality. One day I suddenly realized that I was no longer a 25 year old immortal! I picked up a book on Yoga and read it on the commuter train home. That night I tried my first progressive relaxation session, following the instructions on muscle relaxation in the Yoga book. For me, the relief from all that pent-up stress from my job was indescribable. Many years later when I recall that evening, I still can remember how profound an effect that first session had on me and on the course of my life ever since!

Another benefit of meditation, from the point of view of slowing down the signs of aging, concerns its effects on memory.

Meditation and Memory Research

The myth is that the older you get, the worse your memory and mental abilities become. To the contrary, several studies have shown that those who exercise their minds throughout their lives can actually raise their IQ's! In addition, a recent study found that the memories of people aged 62 to 83 were substantially improved with a program of relaxation training and memory-improvement exercises. If anything will help you stay mentally sharp, meditation will!

Are There Any Drawbacks to Meditation?

Meditation works for most people. Twenty minutes of meditation a day is no more harmful than 20 minutes of prayer. Actually, prayer is a form of meditation. **A WORD OF CAUTION: If you are taking medication for metabolic or endocrine disorders, for psychiatric reasons or for the control of pain, you should be monitored by a physician.** The research findings on meditation report that people who take medication for the above reasons often have their medication reduced and/or eliminated as a result of being involved in a meditation program.

What Are the Most Common Types of Meditation?

Meditation Approach	Mental/Physical Activity
FOCUS ON AN EXTERNAL OBJECT	With your eyes open, you concentrate your attention on an external object which can be almost anything: a candle flame, a painting, the tip of your nose, etc.
FOCUS ON A MENTAL PICTURE	With your eyes closed, you concentrate your attention on a mental picture of a physical object. It can be almost anything, but you would want to avoid an object or picture that upsets you.
FOCUS ON A SPECIFIC BODY PART	With your eyes closed, you concentrate on a specific body part, such as your heart or a point between your eyes sometimes called the "third eye."

Meditation Approach	Mental/Physical Activity
REPEATING A SOUND (Active)	With your eyes closed, you repeat a word or a sound over and over. You concentrate on maintaining the focused state.
REPEATING A SOUND (Passive)	With your eyes closed, you repeat a word or a sound over and over. You make no effort to control your thoughts, and if they wander, you let them. Then, with no effort, go back to repeating the sound.

How Do I Meditate?

Meditation is easier to do than it is to describe. Since it is a very internal personal process, you have to experience it to understand what it can do for you. The rest of the chapter describes the meditation process, step by step. Although meditation is a five-stage process, you can benefit tremendously just from reaching stage three in the chart below.

In a Nutshell, What Is the Meditation Process?

Stages of Meditation	Description
1. **SELECTIVELY PAY ATTENTION**	The first step in meditation is to focus on some thought or object or sound. This means that you are paying attention to only one thing. This is not unlike what happens in a movie theater when the movie comes on and you ignore everything and everyone around you and focus on the colored lights forming objects on the white screen.

In a Nutshell, What Is the Meditation Process?

Stages of Meditation	Description

2. **SUSPEND CRITICAL JUDGMENT**

The second step is that you suspend your critical judgment. Thus, the only reality for you at that moment becomes what your mind is focusing on. This is very similar to the way you behave watching a movie. You temporarily accept the movie as real while you watch it.

3. **HAVE A PHYSICAL RESPONSE**

You begin to have physical responses. The range of physical responses depends on the type of meditation you are practicing. They can range from feeling limp, warm, heavy, etc., to sinking and floating. At this point you should be physically relaxed.

4. **ATTAIN MENTAL CONCENTRATION AND BREATH CONTROL**

The next phase is mental concentration. In this stage you try to calm your mind and to control the flow of your thoughts. This is an inward-focused mode. You can train yourself to remain calm in all situations if you master this art of inward control of the mind. In this state, you allow your thoughts to wander but gently bring yourself back when you catch them wandering. The secret of mastering your thoughts is learning to control your breath.

5. **FLOW TOWARD EFFORTLESS AWARENESS**

The final phase of meditation is an uninterrupted, continuous flow of effortless concentration. This flow is focused on one thought or single point for an extended period of time. In this state, your attention never wavers or wanders. If it is not effortless, if you have to concentrate to stop the flow of thoughts, you are not in the final phase.

TEN BASIC STEPS TO MEDITATING

Meditation Steps	Procedures and Comments

1. **PICK A METHOD**   There are many ways to meditate. Pick up any good Yoga book or a book on meditation and review its suggestions. **You do not need an instructor to learn how to meditate.** However, a good instructor can help you learn ways to meditate and expand your own self-development. There are a number of commercial organizations that charge sizable fees. For the most part, their methods are adaptations of techniques that are available to you in Yoga classes or books. Finding the best way to help you relax quickly depends on your personality. Once you have chosen, stick with the method long enough for it to work. You might also consider using meditation tapes. We have tried a number of them, and based on our own purely subjective responses, we recommend the tapes produced by Martin Brofman, Metavisions, Inc., 130 West 72nd Street, New York, NY 10023. You can also tape your own voice or the voice of someone else using the techniques described at the end of this chapter.

Note from Dave

I prefer to meditate silently without tapes, while Joely prefers the tapes. However, at times when I am feeling tired or extremely stressed, I use tapes as a sort of renewal experience. I especially like tapes on transcontinental flights. It helps to block out the distractions and noise of the jet engines.

Meditation Steps	Procedures and Comments

2. **DON'T MEDITATE ON A FULL STOMACH**

The best times to meditate are when you first wake up, before lunch or dinner, or before you go to bed.

3. **MEDITATE IN A QUIET PLACE**

You must find a quiet place and time to meditate. Psychologically, it is easier to get into the habit of relaxation if you do it at the same time and in the same place every day. The place serves as a psychological cue for your body to relax faster. Whatever distractions there are, don't resist them. Just let them happen. Let the phone ring, ignore the neighborhood kids, etc. Enlist the help of your family, spouse, roommate, children to help you protect your quiet time.

4. **SIT OR LIE DOWN IN A COMFORTABLE POSITION**

An essential part of a successful meditation program is finding a comfortable position in which to meditate. Your back and neck should be straight and your back supported by the chair. Lying flat on the floor is also an excellent position. You can use a small, thin pillow under your head or a rolled-up towel under your neck. A pillow under your knees relieves lower back tension. The whole idea is to find a comfortable position in which you can sit or lie still. Movement interrupts the process.

4a. **Sitting Position**

1) Sit in a comfortable straight-backed chair.

2) Keep your feet flat on the floor and your spine straight.

Meditation Steps	Procedures and Comments

3)   Your hands can be folded on your lap or across your stomach or they can be palms up or palms down in your lap, whatever is most comfortable.

4b.   **Lying Down Position**

1)   Lie flat on your back.

2)   Your head can be flat on the floor or you can place a very thin pillow under it. If you have a neck problem, try putting a tightly rolled towel under your neck. There should be no pressure on the neck area from the towel. Some people are more comfortable with a pillow under their knees.

3)   Hands can be at your sides or folded across your stomach.

5.   **WEAR COMFORT-ABLE CLOTHING**

Get rid of anything that will distract you such as jewelry, tight belts, cuffs, etc. Some people find that wearing the same outfit works the same way as meditating in a special place: the clothing serves as a psychological cue for them to relax.

6.   **KEEP YOUR EYES CLOSED**

For best results, close your eyes. While some people have learned to meditate with their eyes open, most people find that having their eyes closed is the most effective way.

7.   **RELAX YOUR NECK AND BREATHE DEEPLY**

Before beginning meditation, you must learn how to relax your neck and how to breathe deeply. Try performing the following neck and breathing exercises at the beginning of each meditation session.

Meditation Steps	Procedures and Comments
	The purpose of these activities is to help you relax physically so that you can focus your thoughts on your meditation and not be distracted by physical tension. You might think of the breathing and neck exercises as your meditation "warm-up" session.

Visualization for Neck Exercises

It is extremely important that you get your neck muscles relaxed. Visualize as you do these warm-ups that your neck is a piece of warm spaghetti with a heavy ball (your head) hanging from the top. See your neck getting looser and looser as you go through the warm-ups.

7. Head and Neck Warm-ups for Meditation

Step	Illustration

7a. Head forward

1) Sit upright in a low-backed chair with your feet flat on the floor.

2) Tilt your head forward and try to touch your chin to your chest. Relax your neck.

3) Slowly roll your head to an upright position. Repeat three times.

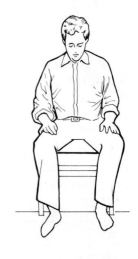

92

Meditation Steps	Illustration

7b. Head backward

1) Sit upright in a low backed chair with your feet flat on the floor.

2) Tilt your head backward and look upward toward the ceiling. Relax your neck.

3) Slowly roll your head to an upright position. Repeat three times.

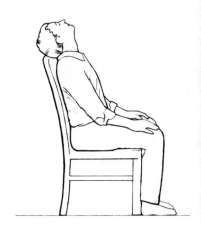

7c. Head sideways

1) Sit upright in a low backed chair with your feet flat on the floor.

2) Tilt your head toward your left shoulder. Try to touch your ear to your shoulder. **Do not lift your shoulder.** Keep your neck relaxed.

3) Slowly return your head to an upright position. Repeat **gently** three times. Then do the same thing on the right side.

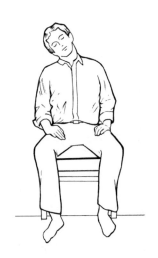

Visualization for Breathing Exercises

In doing the breathing exercises, visualize your belly as a balloon. You want to fill

Meditation Steps **Procedures and Comments**

it up with air when you breathe in and squeeze all the air out of it when you breathe out! As you breathe in, visualize energy and peace filling your body. As you breathe out, visualize all your tiredness and tension flowing out. Feel your muscles relax as you exhale.

Once you have mastered the technique, you will combine it with alternate-nostril breathing. This helps to "center" you and give you a more balanced respiration during meditation.

7. How to Breathe Deeply and Relax

Step **Illustration**

7d. **Fill your lungs**

1) Slowly breathe in. Send the air into your abdomen and feel your stomach expand.

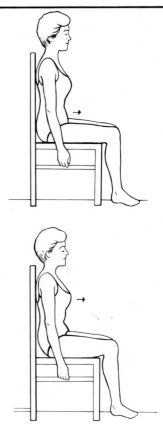

2) Next, fill your lungs and feel your chest expand.

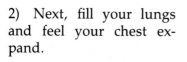

Meditation Steps	Illustration

3) Fill the top of your lungs, pulling your shoulders up to make room for the air.

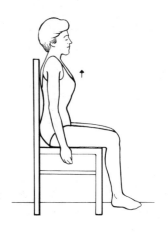

7e. Empty your lungs

1) As you lower your shoulders, slowly empty the top third of your lungs.

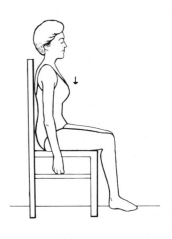

2) Next, push the air slowly out of the middle of your lungs by pulling in your chest.

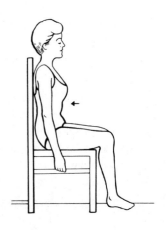

Meditation Steps	Illustration
3) Finally, push your stomach in to force all of the air out of your lungs. Relax.	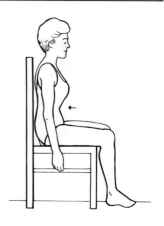

7. How to Relax: Alternate-Nostril Breathing

Step	Illustration
7f. Right-nostril breath 1) Hold your left nostril closed with your index finger. Draw in air through your right nostril. 2) Exhale through your mouth. Repeat three times.	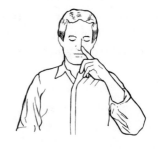
7g. Left-nostril breath 1) Hold your right nostril closed with your index finger. Draw in air through your left nostril. 2) Exhale through your mouth. Repeat three times.	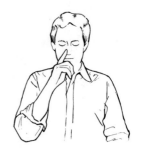

Meditation Steps	Procedures and Comments

8. **MAINTAIN A PASSIVE BUT ALERT ATTITUDE**

The goal is to maintain a passive but alert attitude. Observe your thoughts but don't react. Let them flow through you. You may find all kinds of thoughts going through your mind. Don't resist. Play them out but get a mental picture of their going away. As soon as they are gone, continue meditating. Don't **force** them away. Let them go and quietly start meditating again. If you try to force them from your mind, you'll become tense. Remember, **passive but alert.**

9. **EXPECT TO EXPERIENCE NEW FEELINGS**

Don't be frightened if you experience strange feelings of warmth, color, or electricity running up and down your spine. These are all perfectly natural. Your subconscious will use this time to rid itself of pent-up emotions and sensations. You may even get sexually aroused. It's okay. On the other hand, don't be disappointed if you don't experience any of these sensations.

Some people report extrasensory experiences. We will leave it up to you to decide what these events mean. Prophets and holy men and women from all religions use meditation/prayer as a way to get closer to God. You can incorporate meditation into your religious life to help you experience God more fully. However, you do not have to "believe" in anything to be successful at meditation. Remember, in terms of your health, your purpose is to use meditation as a scientifically established tool to reduce the effects of stress and to help you gain control of your life so that you can stay young, healthy and sexy!

TEN BASIC STEPS TO MEDITATING, continued

Meditation Steps	Procedures and Comments
10. **GO INTO IT SLOWLY AND COME OUT OF IT SLOWLY**	Don't jump up from a meditation session. It's better to return to your normal consciousness slowly. You'll benefit more physically and psychologically.

Can I Start Now?

By all means start now. There's no time like the present. The charts below represent three ways you can meditate. Try them out. Or find sample techniques from other references. The end result will be the same for you regardless of the method you choose.

In this next section there are three separate meditation exercises for you to try out:

1. **An active meditation exercise.**
   In this meditation exercise you will actively guide your mind through a series of visualizations designed to help you relax. You will take a trip to a tropical isle or some other peaceful place of your choice. This type of meditation exercise can help you clarify issues and get a more thorough grasp of the directions you want to go in. There are many versions and variations of active, controlled-thought meditations. A good book on Yoga meditation can supply you with some excellent guided or active meditations for every purpose.

2. **A passive meditation exercise.**
    After you have completely relaxed
    your muscles, you'll repeat a phrase or
    word over and over again, blocking out
    all other thoughts. This procedure is
    very helpful for total relaxation. This
    method has been used for centuries
    and one version has been refined by
    medical scientists.

3. **A healing visualization exercise.**
    In this active meditation exercise you
    will be introduced to a method of vis-
    ualization that has been shown to be
    effective in healing situations.

Note

In all three of the meditation exercises that
follow the first three steps are identical: (1)
neck exercises, (2) alternate nostril breathing, and (3) muscle relaxation. These preliminary steps get you relaxed and ready
for deeper physical and psychological involvement.

AN ACTIVE MEDITATION EXERCISE

Preliminary Step One:
EXERCISE YOUR NECK

Sit in a comfortable chair and do the neck
exercises described previously.

Preliminary Step Two:
DO THE ALTERNATE-NOSTRIL
DEEP BREATHING

Do three or four repetitions of the alternate-nostril breathing exercises described
previously.

Preliminary Step Three:
RELAX YOUR MUSCLES

Lie on your back with your feet spread slightly apart and your arms by your sides. You can lay on a bed, a couch, or the floor, wherever you're comfortable. Hands can be at your sides or resting on your stomach. If you want, put a soft rolled towel or a thin pillow under your neck and a pillow under your knees. Close your eyes and look at an imaginary movie screen between your eyes, sometimes called your mind's eye or the third eye. Tell your mind to banish all negative thoughts. See all of your muscles on the screen. Tell them to relax. Now, shine your mind's "flashlight" on your toes, ask them to relax. Repeat to yourself "My toes are relaxed . . . my toes are relaxed." Continue to shine your flashlight on the various parts of your body, saying "my _____ is relaxed . . . my _____ is relaxed." Start with your toes and work up your body to your feet, ankles, calves, thighs, the whole leg(s), pelvic area, stomach, lower back, shoulders, arms, hands, fingers, upper back, neck, forehead, eyes, lips, tongue. Smooth out all the wrinkles in your forehead. Finally, when you have done every body part, repeat to yourself, "My whole body is relaxed . . . my whole body is relaxed." Feel and experience the deep relaxation. This entire portion of the exercise should not take more than five minutes although you can certainly spend more time on it if you wish.

Note: If you have trouble doing this at first, try tensing your whole body while you inhale. As you exhale, visualize on your "movie screen" your whole body going limp, relaxing. Say to yourself, "I am more relaxed . . . ever more relaxed; my body is getting heavier . . . my body is getting heavier . . . sinking into the floor." With practice, you can learn to relax every muscle in your body at will. The secret is to let go, rather than to command!

CONTROL YOUR BREATHING

Next, concentrate on your breathing. Feel the air enter your nose and move down into your lungs. Listen to it travel back up your windpipe and out your nose. Now, consciously slow down your breathing. As you inhale, see in your mind's eye, and also hear, the word "so." Say to yourself as you inhale, "Soooooooooo . . . ." and as you exhale say, "Hummmmmmmmm . . . ." Use the "so . . . hum" procedure to slow down your breathing. Remember that slowing down the breathing slows down the heart rate and your whole body's rhythm. Let your stomach rise as you inhale and fall back as you exhale. Concentrate on absorbing energy from the air as you inhale and getting rid of stress and nervous energy as you exhale. See yourself in your mind's eye gathering renewed energy as you breath in and out, "soooo . . . hummmm . . . soooo . . . hummmm."

DETACH YOUR MIND

Try to detach your mind. Gently send it away, as far away as you can from your work, your home, your worries, your problems. Visualize some secret and quiet and peaceful place where you would like to be. Only you can go there. Others can come only if you invite them. Travel there in your mind. Visualize yourself actually there. See yourself lying on a beautiful tropical beach for example. Feel yourself travel to your quiet place while you leave your body rest-

101

ing on the floor. When thoughts come to your mind, don't fight them. Accept them gently, and gently banish them. Just watch them go by in your mind as you would watch white clouds passing overhead. Concentrate on keeping your mind blank for a few minutes. Then tell yourself that when you get up you will be extremely well rested and ready for any activity. Now stretch as if you were coming out of a deep sleep and gradually open your eyes. Get up when you're ready.

Time: 10 to 20 minutes

A PASSIVE RELAXATION EXERCISE

EXERCISE YOUR NECK

Sit in a comfortable chair and do the neck exercises described previously.

DO ALTERNATE NOSTRIL DEEP BREATHING

Do three or four repetitions of the alternate nostril breathing exercises described previously.

RELAX YOUR MUSCLES

Do the muscle relaxation exercise previously described.

SELECT A WORD OR PHRASE TO REPEAT

This type of relaxation consists of repeating a word or a phrase over and over. Research shows that it really doesn't matter what the word or phrase is as long as it doesn't create anxiety for you. In other words, don't pick an emotionally loaded word.

I use several phrases. Usually I stick with the same one for six months or even longer. But every once in a while I change. It's a matter of personal preference. You could pick a phrase from your favorite prayer or some other source. I use "I am at peace"; "I am one with the universe", "So . . . hum".

REPEAT YOUR RELAXATION WORD OVER AND OVER

The key to this is making it effortless. Don't force away the thoughts that will enter your mind. Just gently "see" them floating by like white clouds and go back to repeating your phrase "Relax . . . relax" or "I am at peace . . . I am at peace, etc." Some people find that it works better to repeat the phrase only on exhalation. Others just repeat it at their own pace. When you have finished, take the time to reflect on how young and healthy you feel and how joyous it is to re-enter the world having spent these moments at peace with the yourself.
Total Time: 10 to 20 minutes

What About Visualization?

Many people use the "movie screen in their mind" to help them become better performers at almost any task. Visualization is increasingly being used by athletes to help them improve their ability to stay calm in a competitive situation and to enhance their performance. There is considerable scientific evidence that visualization procedures can be extremely useful for such activities. In terms of scientific research on behavior, expectations have been shown to improve performance. Visualizing the expected outcome is an effective technique. You will note that throughout this book wherever we give instructions on how to perform an activity, we have included a visualization where appropriate. Add to or change the visualizations as you like.

A number of people report that visualization helped them heal themselves. Some medical researchers report a great deal of success using visualization/meditation techniques to help speed up the healing process in conjunction with standard medical treatment. There are alternative healing methods that rely exclusively on meditation to heal. Traditional scientists have some difficulty relying only on this approach since they cannot run a lab test or "see" the method actually working. The ability to study directly how the mind "heals" is beyond our technology right now. Yet no one will deny the effect of the mind on health or the possibilities that it offers in the realm of healing. Witness the placebo effect. A well-designed scientific experiment will randomly assign people to two or more groups. The first group will receive some medication or drug that is being tested. The second group will receive a harmless, inactive pill. The placebo effect occurs when people from the second group actually get well because they *think* they are being healed by a drug. Do you have another explanation, besides the power of the mind, for why these people are cured?

A HEALING VISUALIZATION EXERCISE

DEVELOP AN OPTIMISTIC ATTITUDE

Until recently, modern science has pooh-poohed the notion that people can heal themselves with their minds. Recent research has established that it may, in fact, be true. If you are cynical about your ability to make physical changes in your body based on what your mind wills, then don't bother. The self-fulfilling prophecy is never wrong!

EXERCISE YOUR NECK

Sit in a comfortable chair and do the neck exercises described previously.

DO ALTERNATE NOSTRIL DEEP BREATHING

Do three or four repetitions of the alternate nostril breathing exercises described previously.

RELAX YOUR MUSCLES

Do the muscle relaxation exercise previously described.

VISUALIZATION

Close your eyes and look at your "mind's movie screen." See yourself clearly getting younger and perfectly healthy. Look carefully at your face and note that the wrinkles are smoothing out, that your skin is crystal clear and your eyes are sparkling. Hold this mental picture of yourself in your mind. You must see the vision of yourself clearly and in every detail. There is nothing mystical about this process. It's just a focused way of using your imagination. And your imagination is just as powerful an influence on your internal healing mechanism as the stimuli that you take in from your outside reality.

If you want, you can begin saying positive things to yourself like: "Everyday, I'm getting better and better;" "Everyday, I'm getting younger and younger;" "My digestive system is working perfectly;" "I'm very successful," etc.

If there is a particular part of your body that needs work, then picture that body part on your screen, in detail, and see it healing before your eyes. See it in perfect health. Think of your body's defense mechanisms as very strong and the cause of the disease as very weak. See your body easily overcoming the weakness. If you are receiving treatment, see it as very effective and working hand in hand with your body's strong defenses to cure you. Some people actually see their white blood cells as an army conquering the disease. Use your imagination to create a visual picture of yourself achieving perfect health. Any vision that works for you is right.

CHAPTER SEVEN

GOALS AND NOTES FOR RELAXATION

Long Term Relaxation Goal(s)

_____

_____

_____

_____

_____

_____

Short Term Relaxation Goals

_____

_____

_____

_____

_____

_____

_____

_____

_____

_____

_____

Reminder Notes:

_____

_____

_____

_____

_____

_____

NOTES

Social Behavior Of A Long-Life Personality

This chapter will give you a chance to look at yourself from two different perspectives: how you deal with everyday situations, and how you view your rights as a human being interacting with other human beings.

A major characteristic of a long-life personality is knowing how to create constructive relationships that minimize stress and reinforce personal control for both parties. Let's take a look at how you stack up. If you really want to get an interesting look at yourself, have someone close to you rate you on these questions. Write your answers separately, then compare them when the test is completed.

How Do You Deal with Everyday Situations?

Directions: Read each statement, then indicate the degree to which your usual behavior agrees with the statement by circling the appropriate number.

1 = totally disagree
2 = disagree somewhat
3 = undecided or neutral
4 = agree somewhat
5 = totally agree

The Situation	Your Response
1. If someone gets ahead of me in line, I speak up.	Disagree 1-2-3-4-5 Agree
2. At work, I call it the way I see it unless there is obviously no way I can effect a desired change.	Disagree 1-2-3-4-5 Agree
3. If someone doesn't pay me back, I go right up to them and get my money back!	Disagree 1-2-3-4-5 Agree
4. I can say no to anyone.	Disagree 1-2-3-4-5 Agree
5. I tell people, including my relatives, when it is not convenient for me to talk on the phone.	Disagree 1-2-3-4-5 Agree
6. Lots of people get upset when the boss watches them work, but I don't.	Disagree 1-2-3-4-5 Agree
7. The last time someone treated me unfairly, I let him know about it.	Disagree 1-2-3-4-5 Agree
8. When I reflect on it, I'm a pretty good judge of most situations and people.	Disagree 1-2-3-4-5 Agree
9. I only stay late at work when I believe it's necessary and when it doesn't interfere with important personal engagements.	Disagree 1-2-3-4-5 Agree
10. I dispute a bill when I think I have been charged too much, and I don't pay it until the matter has been fully discussed and a mutually acceptable solution has been found.	Disagree 1-2-3-4-5 Agree

The Situation	Your Response

11. If I feel a supervisor has evaluated my performance unfairly, I make an appointment to discuss the matter in detail. The result usually is a change in the evaluation in my favor.

Disagree 1-2-3-4-5 Agree

12. I'm not rude and I try to give other people room to express themselves, but I never ask permission to speak.

Disagree 1-2-3-4-5 Agree

13. I make it a point to get a good table in any restaurant where I am spending my hard-earned money.

Disagree 1-2-3-4-5 Agree

14. I always look for the good in people and have no problem praising their efforts, performance or appearance when it is appropriate.

Disagree 1-2-3-4-5 Agree

15. I always return defective items for exchange or refund regardless of store policy. I am well aware of my rights as a consumer.

Disagree 1-2-3-4-5 Agree

16. I like meeting new people and usually take the initiative in establishing the conversation, but I listen well too.

Disagree 1-2-3-4-5 Agree

The Situation	Your Response

17. I have no problem expressing disagreement, even with people I love or respect.

Disagree 1-2-3-4-5 Agree

18. I never give money to people on the street unless they are from a charitable group to which I normally give.

Disagree 1-2-3-4-5 Agree

19. I believe that hard work is the best way to ensure that you will get what you want from your career.

Disagree 1-2-3-4-5 Agree

20. If I'm waiting to be served and someone who got there after me gets waited on, I immediately speak up.

Disagree 1-2-3-4-5 Agree

TOTAL SCORE: _____

How to Evaluate
Your Personal Control Score

Score Range	Degree of Control
20 – 40	You have little or no control over your life. You are more concerned with what total strangers think of you than with sticking up for yourself.
41 – 55	You have some control, but your life is not very happy because you spend so much time trying to please other people at your own expense.

The Situation	Your Response
56 – 69	You have average control, but your life has no zest.
70 – 79	Not bad, but you could be happier!
80 – 90	You aren't that far from having the total freedom to be yourself!
91 – 100	You're in great shape, and, if you respect other people's rights, you're a wonderful person to deal with!

A person with a long-life personality will resist the manipulations of others, while dealing with others in a non-manipulative way. If you scored lower than you would have liked, don't give up the ship. You were not born to have people walk all over you. Effective social skills are learned, and they can be acquired by anyone. The chart below outlines the social behavior of a long-life personality and shows you which survey items match each characteristic.

Social Behavior of a Long-Life Personality

Characteristic	Behavior
EMOTIONALLY UNINHIBITED	Reveals self freely to others through words and actions. Basic orientation is "What you see is what you get." Survey items #12, 14, 16.
A COMMUNICATOR	Gets along with people from all walks of life. Is open, direct and honest in communicating. Survey items #2, 4, 5, 7, 17.

Characteristic	Behavior
A GO-GETTER	Has an active approach to life. Goes after what he/she wants and usually gets it. Makes things happen. Survey items #11, 13, 19.
HAS SELF-RESPECT	Acts only in ways that increase self-respect. Survey items #1, 3, 10, 15, 20.
INTERNALLY CONTROLLED	Accepts responsibility for own actions. Cannot be manipulated by others and doesn't need to manipulate. Sets and meets goals and is, therefore, exceptionally effective. Survey items #6, 8, 9, 18.

Can I Learn Long-Life Social Skills?

Of course. All social behavior is learned behavior, and you can learn new ways of dealing with people anytime you want. Each time you resist the manipulation of others in specific situations, you free yourself from unnecessary stress. Each time you learn to deal with others in a non-manipulative way, you accomplish the same thing.

All social behavior is learned.

Let's take a look at the attitudes and beliefs you hold about the rules of social interaction so you can figure out where you are. Knowing where you are makes it much easier to know how to get to where you want to go.

Your Inalienable Social Rights
Personal Inventory of Beliefs

Directions: Read each statement and indicate the degree to which you agree with it:

1 = totally disagree
2 = disagree somewhat
3 = undecided or neutral
4 = agree somewhat
5 = totally agree

My Rights	Degree of Agreement about My Rights
1. I can do anything I want to do as long as it is not illegal.	Disagree 1-2-3-4-5 Agree
2. I have the right to say no to anyone at any time.	Disagree 1-2-3-4-5 Agree
3. I have the right to maintain my dignity by asserting myself as long as my purpose is to maintain my dignity and not to put someone else down.	Disagree 1-2-3-4-5 Agree
4. I have the right to say "I don't know" to anyone at any time.	Disagree 1-2-3-4-5 Agree
5. I have the right to make a request of another person at any time as long as I understand that the other person always has the right to say no.	Disagree 1-2-3-4-5 Agree
6. I have the right not to be logical in my decision-making process.	Disagree 1-2-3-4-5 Agree

My Rights	Degree of Agreement about My Rights

7. In social relations there are always gray areas where someone's rights overlap or conflict with mine. In such cases, I have the right to discuss the problem with the person involved so that we can work it out.

Disagree 1-2-3-4-5 Agree

8. I have the right to say "I don't understand" to anyone at any time.

Disagree 1-2-3-4-5 Agree

9. I have the right to maintain my rights even if someone else gets hurt.

Disagree 1-2-3-4-5 Agree

10. I am the best judge of my own behavior, emotions, feelings and opinions.

Disagree 1-2-3-4-5 Agree

11. I have the right to say "I don't care" to anyone at any time.

Disagree 1-2-3-4-5 Agree

12. I have the right to take responsibility for my own behavior, feelings and thoughts and to deal with the consequences.

Disagree 1-2-3-4-5 Agree

13. I have the right to judge whether or not I want to be responsible for helping others solve thier problems.

Disagree 1-2-3-4-5 Agree

14. I have the right not to offer reasons or excuses for my behavior.

Disagree 1-2-3-4-5 Agree

My Rights	Degree of Agreement about My Rights
15. I have the right to make mistakes.	Disagree 1-2-3-4-5 Agree
16. I have the right to be responsible for my errors.	Disagree 1-2-3-4-5 Agree
17. I have the right to be free of the good opinion of other people when I deal with them. This means that I do not have to work at getting them to like me. I can work at maintaining my rights.	Disagree 1-2-3-4-5 Agree
18. I have the right to change my mind anytime I want to.	Disagree 1-2-3-4-5 Agree

Total Score: _____

How to Determine Your Understanding of Your Inalienable Social Rights

Score	Degree of Understanding
90	You fully understand your rights and need only make certain that you have the appropriate social skills to defend and maintain them while allowing other people their rights.
72-89	You have a pretty good grasp of your rights but have not yet learned that there is no compromise on social rights or freedoms.
54-71	You have a great deal to learn about your rights. No doubt there are many times when you are unhappy about social situations where you have allowed people to

Score	Degree of Understanding
	deprive you of your rights out of some misguided notion of fairness or fear of loss of love. You need to reexamine what you have learned about social interactions in light of the fact that everyone, including you, has these inalienable rights.
18-53	People walk all over you. Many times you're angry in social situations and you can't even figure out why you resent such interactions.

If you are not used to thinking about social interactions in terms of rights, the statements you read may seem rather strident to you. However, when they are put into operation by someone with a long-life personality, they are not in the least bit harsh or strident. They give you and the other person complete freedom to act as equals and to jointly create a constructive relationship that minimizes stress and reinforces personal control for both of you. Even when you're the only one in the interaction who is operating under these principles, they allow you to free yourself from other people's manipulations and to be non-manipulative in your own dealings. The next two chapters give some examples of how you can implement these rights in your own life.

CHAPTER EIGHT WORKSHEET

Long Term Goal(s)_____ Rewards _____

_____

_____

_____

_____

_____

_____

_____

_____

_____

Short Term Goals _____ Rewards _____

_____

_____

_____

_____

_____

_____

_____

_____

_____

Reminder Notes: _____

_____

_____

_____

_____

NOTES

The Psychology Of Interpersonal Relations

Our interactions with other people are often the greatest source of stress in our lives. It doesn't have to be that way. There are ways of dealing with people that enhance the self-esteem of both parties and actually reduce stress. Chapter 8 gave you an opportunity to rate yourself in your everyday dealings with other people. It also gave you the chance to see how comfortable you feel with your basic interpersonal rights. Now that you've taken stock of where you are, it's time to start looking at where you want to go and how to get there.

This chapter will teach you:

The things in life that can't be changed and aren't worth worrying about.

Four basic principles for interpersonal relationships.

SEVEN THINGS IN LIFE THAT CAN'T BE CHANGED
And Therefore Are Not Worth Worrying About

You Can't Change:	Face It Now

---

1. **YOUR FAMILY HISTORY AND UPBRINGING**	You can't change the way your parents dealt with you. You can't change the fact that your brother/sister was the favorite child or that you were picked on, etc. These are things of the past. Accept them and get on with your life.

You Can't Change:	Face It Now
2. **YOUR VITAL STATISTICS**	No doubt you can improve your looks with hair color, wigs, caps on your teeth and plastic surgery if you are very determined, but for the most part you can't change your basic physical characteristics. This book is about self-development. In order to change yourself so that you can stay young, healthy and sexy, you must accept those things about yourself that you cannot change and concentrate on those things you can change.
3. **OTHER PEOPLE**	People will live their own lives their own way and you can't change that fact. Accept it and stop worrying about it.
4. **FATHER TIME**	Time marches on and there's nothing you can do to stop it.
5. **MOTHER NATURE**	You can't change the weather, but you can make each day a happy one regardless of it!
6. **HISTORY**	The South lost the Civil War. Napoleon was defeated at Waterloo. What's past is past and you can't change it. What happened to you, your loved ones, your friends, your enemies can't be undone. The past is only good for the lessons you can learn from it. Once you have learned the lesson, close the book and think about now!
7. **DEATH AND TAXES**	Although death is inevitable, how you get there is up to you. You can live the average sendentary life-style. You can eat the average high-protein high-fat low-fiber diet. You can condemn yourself to increased illness and medical bills and a concurrent decline in the quality of your life. Or you can choose to do something for yourself. It's entirely up to you.

Once you stop worrying about things you can't change, you free up a tremendous amount of energy to do something about the things that you can change. Changing the way you deal with people can have tremendous payoff for both you and them. Below are four basic principles for interpersonal relations that are part of the long-life personality.

Four Principles of Interpersonal Relations

Principle	Description
1. **I CANNOT CHANGE OTHER PEOPLE'S BEHAVIOR, I CAN ONLY CHANGE MY OWN BEHAVIOR.**	How many times have you said, "If only so and so would change, everything would be different," or "If only my boss would let me know when I've done a good job, I would be more motivated in work." Those kinds of statements put all the responsibility on the other person. If you have a long-life personality, you take responsibility for your half of the relationship.
	As human beings we are social animals. We respond to stimuli. If you don't like what is going on in a relationship, you need to think about the stimulus you are presenting. If the stimulus brings out behavior you don't like, you need to change the stimulus. You can't sit around and wait for the other person to change his or her behavior, because it won't happen. If you continue to present the same stimulus, the other person will continue to respond with the same behavior. If you change the stimulus, the response will change.
	What do you think would happen if you went to your boss and said something like, "I'm feeling a little discouraged. I don't get

any feedback from you on my projects. I think I did a real good job, but hearing something from you would help me evaluate my performance." Don't you think your boss would become more aware that she needs to increase her feedback to staff? But you can't sit around and moan about lack of feedback; you have to change your own behavior first if you want the other person to change his or her behavior.

2. **YOU TEACH PEOPLE TO TREAT YOU THE WAY THEY DO.**

Do you let your children treat you as a free babysitting service...and then resent it? Do you let your neighbor continue to send her kids to your house after school even though you're beginning to hate the sight of them? Do you let your boss believe that you're available to work late and on Saturdays without any notice while you smile on the outside and seethe on the inside? People treat you the way you teach them to treat you. If you want someone to treat you differently, you have to take the initiative to change your behavior and teach them to treat you differently.

You have to tell people how you feel; they can't read your mind. Have you hesitated to say anything because you're afraid of hurting the other person's feelings? That's a real copout. Be honest with yourself. You're not afraid of hurting her feelings. You're afraid she won't like/love you any more. Imagine telling this person how you really feel. Imagine this person telling you that she's really glad you said something...that she's wanted to change the situation for some time but thought you would be upset. What a relief! The real reason you don't say anything is that you're afraid she'll be angry with you, or she'll think you're selfish, or she won't talk to you any more.

People treat you the way you teach them to treat you. The next time your daughter drops by with the kids, you can be really truthful and tell her that you've paid your dues and that you want to enjoy the free time that you have worked so hard to have. If you can't bring yourself to be so blunt, tell her that you wish you could help but you have other plans. If you do this often enough, she will be forced to make other arrangements because you will have taught her by your actions that you are not always available. You can do the same with your neighbor.

Do you really think your boss would fire you if you told him that you have a commitment that can't be changed on such short notice? Remember, you can't expect other people to change their behavior if you don't make the effort to change yours.

3. **YOU CHOOSE TO FEEL AND REACT THE WAY YOU DO.**

"It makes me so upset that I have to lie down." Your feelings are not forced on you from the outside. They are there because you choose to have them. There is always an emotional payoff for any feeling. If you want to change your feelings, you need to find out what your payoff is. It's possible that you choose to be upset because you found on previous occasions that it gets you attention. Being upset may also mean that other people take care of the problem for you when you're "too upset" to do it yourself. You get to lie down and someone else gets to clean up the problem. What a deal!

Guilt is another insidious emotion. We often choose to feel guilty rather than admit that we really don't want to do something. We also choose to feel guilty as a way of convincing ourselves that we're nice people even though we didn't do such and such. How many times have you felt guilty about not calling someone? Let's face it: if you really wanted to call that person, you would. You would make the time. You're choosing to feel guilty as a way of telling yourself that you still care about that person even though you don't want to talk to him/her right now.

Face up to the reality of your emotions and why you choose to have them. Life is much more exciting when you, and not your emotions, are in control.

4. **TREAT OTHER PEOPLE THE WAY YOU WANT THEM TO TREAT YOU.**

The golden rule goes back beyond written history. It has been an operating principle for every religion in the world. Why? Because it works. It is the logical extension of the first two principles we discussed: *You can't change other people's behavior, you can only change your own;* and *you teach people to treat you the way they do.*
Just think about the last time someone did something nice for you without being asked. How did you feel towards that person? Warm? Friendly? Did you want to reciprocate? Of course you did. It's human nature to respond in kind. If you're mean to me, I'll be mean to you. If you're nice to me, I'll be nice to you. It's normal to want to be around people who treat you with respect. So start now and begin to treat with respect everyone with whom you deal. Treat them the way you want to be treated. It's bound to come back to you.

Now that you've had an overview of the four operating principles, here are some strategies for implementing them.

Strategies for Implementing Principle No. 1

I CAN'T CHANGE OTHER PEOPLE'S BEHAVIOR, I CAN ONLY CHANGE MY OWN

---

1. **FIGURE OUT WHAT YOU ARE DOING THAT ELICITS THE UNDESIRED RESPONSE.**

   Example 1
   Your kids are driving you crazy because they don't pick up their clothes and you end up doing it. Obviously, your behavior of picking up the clothes elicits their response of ignoring your requests. They have learned that they don't have to pick up their clothes. If they procrastinate long enough, you'll do it.

   Example 2
   Even though you've told your husband that you're on a diet, he buys you candy. The fact that you eat the candy reinforces his belief that you aren't serious.

2. **DECIDE ON A DIFFERENT WAY OF DEALING WITH THE PROBLEM.**

   In the example of the kids, you need to change your behavior. An obvious solution is to stop picking up their clothes. If they have to wear dirty, wrinkled clothes several days in a row, they'll learn to pick up their clothes. What's that you say? Your kids couldn't care less about wrinkles in their clothes? Then your approach could be to refuse to serve them dinner until they pick up their clothes. If they really believe that you'll let them go hungry, they'll pick up their clothes in a hurry.

   In the second example, you need to stop eating the candy. If you find it impossible to have it in the house without eating it, then open up the box and throw the individual pieces in the garbage. Or walk across

127

the street and give it to your neighbor. Make sure you tell your husband that you love him for thinking about you, but that roses or a new book or new running shorts would have been a perfect gift because you are on a diet and it's very difficult for you to have self-control when you can smell chocolate from 50 yards away.

3. **IF THE SITUATION WARRANTS IT, TELL THE PEOPLE INVOLVED WHAT BEHAVIOR YOU EXPECT AND WHAT YOU WILL DO IF YOU DON'T GET IT.**

Once you tell people what you will do, *make sure you do it!*

Strategies for Implementing Principle No. 2

YOU TEACH PEOPLE TO TREAT YOU THE WAY THEY DO

1. **FIGURE OUT WHAT EXACTLY YOU'RE TEACHING PEOPLE.**

Your five-year-old daughter wants to watch television while she eats. You say no. She says, "Please, please." You say no louder. She starts to whine. You say that you'll spank her if she doesn't stop. She stops for a little while and then starts again, even more loudly. You spank her, feel guilty and turn on the TV. What have you taught her? You've taught her that if she is willing to put up with a little yelling and a spanking, she can have what she wants. You've also taught her that you don't necessarily mean it when you say no, and if she persists long enough, you may change your mind.

2. **IMPLEMENT PRINCIPLE NO. 1 AND CHANGE YOUR BEHAVIOR.**

Decide on a different approach when she starts to whine. You might say, "In this house we don't watch TV while we eat. We talk to each other about our day. If you don't want to talk to us, you can leave the table." If she chooses to leave the table and go hungry, let her do it. Just make sure you don't feed her later on in the evening or you will be teaching her an entirely different lesson.

3. **REINFORCE THE DESIRED BEHAVIOR.**

It's important for you to let people know that you like their new behavior. Tell your kids that you really like it when they pick up their clothes. Let your husband know that the running shorts were absolutely perfect and that you feel really good when he supports you in your weight loss program. Tell your daughter that you really like it when she sits at the table like a grown-up and participates in the discussion.

Strategies for Implementing Principle No. 3

YOU CHOOSE TO FEEL AND REACT THE WAY YOU DO

1. **FIGURE OUT WHAT THE EMOTIONAL PAYOFF IS FOR WHAT YOU'RE FEELING**

Are you choosing to feel angry instead of doing something about it? Anger is a perfectly valid emotion, but after you acknowledge that you're angry, you should be thinking about how you will change your behavior so that the situation doesn't happen again.

Are you choosing to feel guilty in order to convince yourself that you really are a loving parent, child, spouse, friend?

2. **REREAD THE LIST OF SOCIAL RIGHTS IN CHAPTER 8.** After you've reread the list of rights, read it again, and again. You're a nice person whether you call your friend or not. You're a loving parent whether you lose your temper or not.

Strategies for Implementing Principle No. 4

TREAT OTHER PEOPLE THE WAY YOU WANT THEM TO TREAT YOU

1. **TREAT OTHERS WITH RESPECT** You don't have to agree with people in order to show respect for their social rights. You only have to grant them the list of rights discussed in Chapter 8.

2. **LISTEN** Let other people talk. Genuinely pay attention. Use the information that they give you about themselves to improve the relationship.

3. **GIVE CREDIT** Whenever you are working with someone, make sure you give them credit for their share in the success of the project.

4. **PUT ON THEIR SHOES** Try to see the other person's point of view. You don't have to agree with their position, but it helps in making decisions about how best to interact with them when you see where they are coming from.

5. **ADMIT IT WHEN YOU'RE WRONG** When you are wrong, admit it. Honesty is very disarming. (Things might have gone differently for Richard Nixon had he followed this strategy!)

When you apply the interpersonal strategies suggested for the four principles, it is very helpful to be aware of the way you communicate. You may very well be using the correct words and not be delivering the message that you expected. Body posture, eye contact, tone, etc., are all part of the true message that you are sending the other person. The techniques below will help you show others that you are a strong, self-confident and dynamic person.

Seven Communication Skills That Make You Look Strong, Self-Confident and Dynamic

Communication Approach	Technique
1. **EYE CONTACT**	Look directly at the person with a relaxed steady gaze. Do not look away from the person or down.
2. **BODY POSTURE**	Sit opposite the person rather than beside him. Sit erect and lean towards him.
3. **GESTURES**	Use relaxed hand and arm gestures but don't overdo them. Control nervous gestures, but don't keep your hands at your sides or on your lap.
4. **FACIAL EXPRESSION**	Practice having a pleasant facial expression in the mirror. If you frown when you are saying something nice, the message is clear that you are angry or worried. If you smile when you are angry, the message that you are angry does not come across.
5. **VOICE TONE, VOLUME, INFLECTION**	Your voice should be well-modulated. Audio-tape your voice and listen. Practice not being too soft, too loud or boring.

6. **FLUENCY**   Speak slowly, smoothly. If you talk too quickly or show hesitation, you come across as unsure.

7. **POSITIVE CONTENT**   Express what you feel honestly in accordance with the list of social rights. Keep your statements positive and don't put other people down.

How Do I Learn to Use These Techniques?

Chapters 8 and 9 have provided you with a number of strategies for improving your interpersonal skills. In order to learn how to use them, you must practice, practice, practice. Enlist the help of a loved one or friend to help you act out different scenes. Try the techniques out, one at a time, and rehearse them. Don't get upset if they don't work the first time. Review, analyze, start again. **Master one technique at a time.** The chart below outlines the process you should follow for learning new techniques.

THE EIGHT STEPS TO LEARNING NEW SOCIAL BEHAVIOR

1. **FIND OUT WHERE YOU ARE NOW**   Make an assessment of where you are now by observing your own behavior. Be your own fly on the wall. After an event, reflect on what happened and think about it. Were you effective? What could you have done to make it work better?

2. KEEP TRACK

Keep a record of your progress. Look for patterns of success or failure.

3. WORK ON ONE THING AT A TIME

If you try to master more than one social skill at a time you will have difficulty. Practical experience and research have shown that it is faster and easier to learn one step at a time.

4. VISUALIZE

Research has shown that if you mentally rehearse what you plan to do, your actual performance will be better and smoother. Relax and see yourself handling the situation calmly, smoothly, easily.

5. CRITIQUE YOURSELF

After each event, critique yourself. Compare yourself to where you were in step 1 above. Make a list of the things you said or did correctly and a list of things that did not work for you. Make a list of ways you think you can improve your performance when a similar situation occurs.

6. FIND A ROLE MODEL

If at all possible, find someone who does very well what you are trying to learn. Watch him or her operate.

7. GET FEEDBACK

Seek out feedback from friends and others who are willing to tell you how you handled the situation. If you have found a "pro," get him or her to give you feedback.

8. REWARD YOURSELF

The key to success in any behavior-modification plan is reward. It doesn't have to be a material reward to work. It can be almost anything as long as it's something you like. Every time you successfully make an attempt to stand up for one of your social rights, make sure there is a reward at the end for you!

CHAPTER NINE WORKSHEET

Long Term Goal(s) _____ Rewards _____

_____

_____

_____

_____

_____

_____

_____

Short Term Goals _____ Rewards _____

_____

_____

_____

_____

_____

_____

_____

_____

_____

Reminder Notes: _____

_____

_____

_____

_____

_____

_____

_____

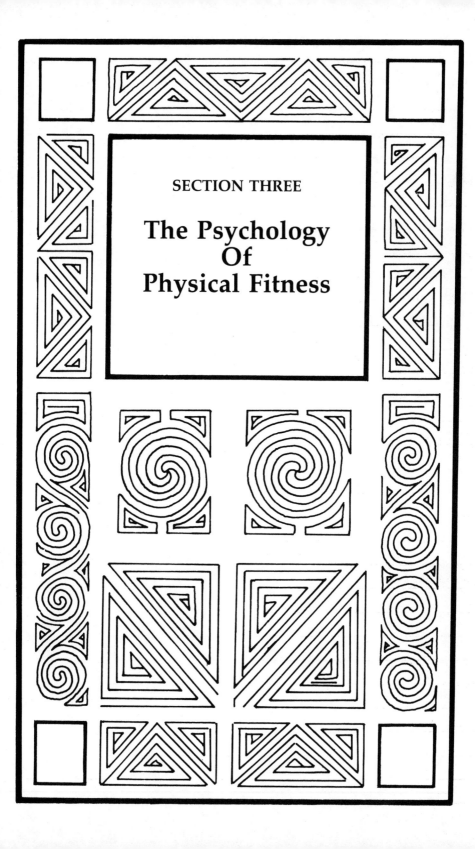

SECTION THREE

The Psychology
Of
Physical Fitness

Choosing
An Aerobic Program

What Is Aerobics and Why Should I Care?

An aerobic activity is any kind of body movement that requires you to use a lot of oxygen over a sustained period of time. The ability of your body to handle oxygen under this kind of stress is called its vital capacity, a powerful predictor of longevity. There is increasing scientific evidence that people who exercise aerobically have fewer chronic illnesses and, in particular, a significantly reduced risk of cardiovascular disease. Aerobics also has a number of other benefits.

Scientifically Established Benefits of Aerobics

PHYSICAL BENEFITS OF AEROBICS

* Heart muscles become thicker and stronger.

* Pulse rate slows down.

* Blood pressure drops.

* Red blood cells increase.

* Energy increases.

* Digestion improves.

* Bowels function better.

* Appetite is brought into line with your body's needs.

* Weight loss is accelerated.

* Sex drive increases.

* Body temperature rises by several degrees while exercising, which helps to kill bacteria.

* The level of high-density lipoproteins (HDL) increases. HDL help to keep fat from building up in the arteries.

* The body is more sensitive to insulin, a real benefit to diabetics.

* With running in particular, calcium loss in bones is prevented, which guards against osteoporosis, a crippling bone disease. Osteoporosis starts around age 35. Thirty percent of women and 10% of men over 60 suffer from it, and 50% of all people over 70 have it.

PSYCHOLOGICAL BENEFITS OF AEROBICS

* Helps control depression.

* Reduces stress.

* Improves self-concept.

* Increases mental productivity.

* Improves problem-solving skills.

What Do I Do First?

It is essential that you have a physical examination and a stress test for your heart. We recommend that the physical be given by a physician who is in good physical condition!

What Do I Do Next?

Determine your exercise heart rate (EHR). The whole idea of aerobics is to get your heart rate high enough to force your cardiovascular system to make beneficial physical changes.

WARNING: Do not start an aerobics program without your physician's approval and without having had a complete physical examination.

Your physician should be able to help you determine the heart rate at which you'll want to function when you begin your aerobic program, or you can try your local health club, university sports-medicine department or similar organization. They will be able to either provide the service or refer you to a place that can.

One alternative, if you are in excellent health, is to do it yourself using the formula suggested by Dr. Kenneth H. Cooper, the "dean" of aerobics:

Formulas For Calculating Exercise Heart Rate (EHR) for Your Aerobic Activity

Formula for Men:

EHR = 220 minus age X .80

Example: Dave is 50 years old. His exercise heart rate is calculated as follows:

Dave's EHR = 220-50 X .80 = 136

$$EHR = 205 - (age/2) \; X \; .80$$

Example: Joely is 37 years old. Her exercise heart rate is calculated as follows:

Joely's EHR $= 205-(37/2) \; X \; .80 = 149$

How To Take Your Own Pulse

You can feel your pulse at your wrist or by putting your hand over your heart. Count the number of beats for 15 seconds and multiply by four.

Implementing the 3% Formula for Aerobics

Now that you have determined what your desired exercise heart rate is, you need to begin an aerobic program that will get your heart working at that rate for a minimum of 20 minutes per day at least four days per week. You can get all the mental and physical benefits of aerobics in only 1 hour and 20 minutes per week. That's only a little over 1% of the total time you have available to you in a week. Even if you add dressing time and a five-minute cool down, you are still well under 2% of your time per week.

Fitting It Into Your Schedule

People who work have basically three choices of when they will do their aerobic exercise: in the morning, at a club during lunch, or in the evening before dinner. Research has shown that running before dinner suppresses the appetite, speeds up the metabolic process and increases weight loss. Personally, we have found that we get too involved in our work to stop and get ready to run. When we've said that we're going to run before dinner, we never seem to do it, so we make a point of running in the morning. That way, we make sure we get it in. Although it's absolutely true that you have to get up earlier in the morning, it's also true that regular aerobic exercise increases your energy level. In the long run, the benefits of aerobic activity far outweigh the effort that goes into doing it.

A Note from Joely

Our weekend schedule runs a little later than our weekday schedule. We have David's two children on the weekends and we often let them ride their bikes along-side us while we run. It's a good way to get them involved, and we feel we're providing positive role models for them.

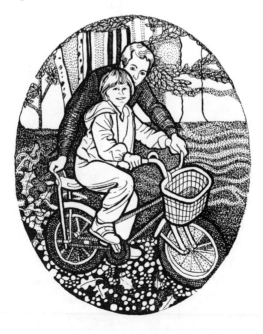

Nine Steps To A Successful Aerobic Program
A Psychological Approach

1. **PICK THE BEST TIME**

    Psychologically, if you don't pick a time that is most convenient, you will not stick to the program. You'll come up with a dozen excuses not to exercise based on bad timing. Consider both your personal and business schedule. Walking could take too much out of your daily schedule if you have to commute long hours. Swimming may present a problem if the local pool hours are in conflict with your schedule or if the club is too far from home, etc.

2. **PICK TWO ALTERNATIVES**

    Another way for you to cop out is to find a reason not to follow your aerobic schedule because of the weather or some other factor (e.g., can't bike, it's snowing; can't run, it's raining; can't swim, the pool is being drained, etc.). Therefore, we recommend that you pick two aerobic activities because this gives you options. For example, if you're a runner and it's icy out, you can still swim. Having two aerobic alternatives also cuts down on the risk of boredom, another factor that your marvelous mind can use in making up excuses for you not to exercise.

3. **TAKE IT SLOW AND EASY**

    If you try to achieve your aerobic goals too fast, you not only run the risk of injury, you also run the psychological risk of becoming discouraged. Work up to fitness gradually. As you meet each short-term fitness goal, you will be more motivated to continue.

4. **WRITE DOWN YOUR PROGRAM GOALS**

    Psychologically, you are more likely to stick with an aerobic program if you write down your goals, with times, days of the weeks, etc. Many people need charts, graphs,

142

targets, etc., to motivate themselves. Buy the best-selling books on the activities you have chosen and work out a program. There are even software programs available for those who want to print out graphs and charts of daily progress!

5. **MAKE YOUR NEW HABIT A REGULAR HABIT**

Whether you need charts or not, be consistent in your program. Do it regularly every chosen day at the same time. This way you will become psychologically and physiologically accustomed to the routine. Eventually, with practice, your aerobic workout will become as habitual to you as brushing your teeth. Don't skip more than one day. It's much too easy, particularly in the beginning, to go back to your old ways of sedentary nonactivity.

6. **CHOOSE A MEASURABLE AEROBIC ACTIVITY**

The psychological reason for making your primary aerobic activity one that is measurable is that you must be able to "see" progress if you expect to stay motivated. Remember that your stiff and worn-out body will try everything it can to persuade you not to exercise! Your job is to get that same body physically fit so that it will protest when you don't exercise!

There are other ways to get aerobically fit besides the ones we recommend, but they're difficult to quantify. For example, it's easy to quantify running by time and distance; it's not easy to quantify aerobic dancing, or tennis or racquetball. Use them as your secondary or alternate aerobic exercise.

7. **DON'T GET COMPETITIVE**

We do not recommend competitive physical activities for most people. One of the benefits of an aerobic program is the reduction of stress and stress-related symptoms. Why add another competitive situation to your already stressful life?

8. **HAVE FUN DOING IT!**

We have included one activity in our recommended group for which we do not offer monitoring charts or suggestions. This is cross-country skiing. It is probably the best all around aerobic activity; however, it is not something you can do year-round. We cross-country ski for the fun of it and skip our regular running/swimming routine on that day!

9. **REWARD YOURSELF**

Without rewards, any behavior modification program is doomed to failure. For each increment or short-term goal that is achieved have a planned reward set up well in advance. Remember, don't pick a reward that is in conflict with your goals. Psychological rewards are usually more effective than material ones. Joely just rewarded herself by attending her 20th high school reunion. It's a terrific boost to your morale to discover that you are still as trim and toned as you were in high school while many of your classmates look old enough to be your mother or father!

Running/Jogging

A lot of running aficionados like to make distinctions between running and jogging. Jogging has been defined as bouncing up and down as you move at a walking pace. Others say you are running only when you can make a mile in less than nine minutes. In our opinion, any normal human being can see the difference between a person who is walking and one who is running. Speed is irrelevant. It's how you use your body that makes the distinction.

Positive Checklist for Running

---

* It doesn't require special equipment, just a good pair of running shoes.

* There are lots of books on running that you can read.

* You don't need to go to any special place to run – just pick any street.

* You can run alone or be social and run with others.

* It can be competitive or not – your choice.

* It's easy to measure change, development, and growth.

* There are no skill requirements.

* Running in particular guards against osteoporosis by contributing to stronger bones.

Aerobic Ratings for Running/Jogging

Pace Of Activity	Calories Burned 20 mins.	30 mins.	Aerobic Rating
Running 1 mile in 12 mins.	160	240	High

Pace Of Activity	Calories Burned 20 mins.	30 mins.	Aerobic Rating
Running 1 mile in 11 mins.	200	300	High
Running 1 mile in 10 mins.	220	330	High

Drawbacks to Running

The single biggest drawback to running is the risk of injury. One way to avoid injury is to warm up properly. There is some controversy over what this means. A recent study found that those who stretched too much before running were more prone to injury. For warm-ups we recommend the knee-to-chest exercises discussed in the chapter following this one, plus running slower than an eight-minute mile for the first mile.

The critical activity, in our opinion, is stretching **after** the run. For cooling down, we do a five minute walk and a 20-to-30 minute flexibility routine. See the next chapter for the stretching/flexibility program.

Another drawback to running is the pounding your body takes. While this accounts for the fact that your bones get stronger as a result of running, it does have an effect on joints. Good running shoes go a long way toward minimizing the problem. You can also run on a padded track.

The way to minimize the risk of injury and at the same time improve performance is to learn how to use your body more efficiently and with ease. A very good method which we have recently been studying and applying to our everyday activities is called the Alexander Technique. While the technique has much broader application than its use in aerobic activities, we feel that this is an appropriate point to introduce it because of its ability to reduce the risk of injury while performing vigorous physical activities.

The Alexander Technique

If you ask someone who has taken Alexander lessons to describe the experience, most would be hard pressed to put it into words. That's because the Alexander Technique has to be experienced to be fully understood. Over 25 years of research, much of it conducted at the Tufts University Institute for Experimental Psychology, plus an enormous amount of accumulated clinical information over many years lend support to the success of the technique in helping people to (1) learn to release chronic physical tensions, (2) improve spinal alignment and posture, (3) improve muscular coordination, (4) improve muscle tone and (5) get rid of unconscious but unwanted muscle responses to physical and emotional stimuli and to substitute new, more healthy physical, mental and emotional responses.

The technique was discovered and developed at the turn of the century by F. Matthias Alexander, an Australian actor who kept losing his voice. Unable to get help from traditional sources, Alexander began to study himself with mirrors. He discovered that when he began to speak in public he put downward pressure on his spine by moving his head backward and downward. He developed a method to inhibit himself from doing this. In the process, he soon discovered the enormous potential of learning to "use the self," as he called it, in a different and more effective way. Eventually, this led to the Alexander Technique, an organized method for controlling and changing physical responses and reactions and substituting more appropriate ones.

While very few people have been able to learn the Alexander Technique on their own, the beauty of the system is that the goal of the instruction is to teach you how to do it yourself without a teacher!

A number of prominent figures earlier in the century were proponents of the technique, including Aldous Huxley, George Bernard Shaw and John Dewey. Dewey, the famous educational philosopher, began his lessons at age 58. He attributed much of the rejuvenation and vigor that followed for the next 35 years of his life to the technique. More recently, Professor Nikolaas Tinbergen, the winner of the Nobel Prize for Medicine in 1973, and his family studied the Alexander Technique. He gave a major address and wrote an article about it noting, among other things, that the impact of the technique had been a profound one in terms of the mental and physical well-being of his family.

In spite of the research, clinical data and the involvement of prominent people, the Alexander Technique has remained, until recently, a well-kept secret in the United States. We recommend that those who are participating in vigorous physical activities consider taking Alexander

Technique lessons to help improve their ability to move freely under stress and thus minimize the risk of injury. As we have learned to apply the Alexander principles in running and swimming, we've found that we really don't need to warm up. It has also made it possible for us to gain greater benefits from our flexibility training. As we progress, we find that it helps us with our meditation too.

You can find out about Alexander teachers in your area by contacting the Alexander Technique Association of New England, 15A Channing Street, Cambridge, MA 02138 (617-497-2242) or the American Center for the Alexander Technique, 142 West End Avenue, New York, NY 10023 (212-799-0468) or the F.M. Alexander Technique Workshops, P.O. Box 408, Ojai, CA 93023.

Your Personal Start-Up Plan

We've included two start-up plans: one for people under 30 and one for people over 30. We've also included time for a flexibility/stretching program to follow your running. Running tightens your muscles. You need to stretch and flex them in order to keep them loose. We can attest to the benefits of a flexibility program from personal experience. As a result of a flexibility program, Dave had absolutely no stiffness when he began running. Joely had only minor soreness in her Achilles tendons, which is a small miracle for someone who has worn high heels every day of her adult life.

PERSONAL START-UP PLAN FOR RUNNING
(Healthy, Under 30)

WEEKLY GOALS

Step	What To Do	Times Per Week	Miles	Minutes Per Mile	Cool Down (Mins.)	Flexi- bility* (Mins.)	Total Hrs:Mins. Per Wk.
1	walk	3	2.0	15	n/a	20	2:30
2	walk	3	3.0	15	n/a	20	3:15
3	walk/run	4	2.0	13	5	20	3:24
4	walk/run	4	2.0	12	5	20	3:16
5	run	4	2.0	11	5	20	3:08
6	run	4	2.0	10	5	20	3:00
7	run	5	2.0	10	5	20	3:45
8	run	4	2.5	10	5	20	3:20
9	run	4	2.5	9.5	5	20	3:15
10	run	4	3.0	9	5	20	3:28

*Note: See the next chapter for step-by-step directions for a flexibility program. We recommend a 20-minute flexibility program five days a week, so you'll be doing additional flexibility training on days when you do not do aerobic exercise.

If you are over 30, you may want to go a little slower than the plan above. The next chart contains a personal start-up program for those who are healthy and over 30.

PERSONAL START-UP PLAN FOR RUNNING
(Healthy, Over 30)

WEEKLY GOALS

Step	What To Do	Times Per Week	Miles	Minutes Per Mile	Cool Down (Mins.)	Flexi-bility* (Mins.)	Total Hrs:Mins. Per Wk.
1	walk	3	2.0	17	n/a	20	2:42
2	walk	3	2.5	17	n/a	20	3:08
3	walk	3	3.0	16.5	n/a	20	3:29
4	walk/run	4	2.0	13.00	5	20	3:24
5	walk/run	4	2.0	12.00	5	20	3:16
6	run	4	2.0	11.00	5	20	3:08
7	run	4	2.0	10.00	5	20	3:00
8	run	5	2.0	10.00	5	20	3:45
9	run	4	2.5	10.00	5	20	3:20
10	run	4	3.0	10.00	5	20	3:40

*Note: See the next chapter for step-by-step directions for a flexibility program. We recommend a 20-minute flexibility program five days a week, so you'll be doing additional flexibility training on days when you do not do aerobic exercise.

Swimming

Swimming is probably the best all around aerobic exercise. It exercises the upper and lower body at the same time. The forces of gravity are held in check in the water, thus practically eliminating the risk of injury and the wear and tear on joints and tendons. On top of all these benefits, swimming is a "no sweat" activity. Your body cools 25 times faster in water than it does in air...so, even though you're working hard, it doesn't really feel like it!

Positive Checklist for Swimming

---

* Involves all major muscles in activity.

* Less risk of injury than any other aerobic activity.

* Less strain on joints and bones.

* Lots of social opportunities at poolside.

* Can be competitive or not, as desired.

* Can be combined with other activities such as scuba diving, beach parties, etc.

Aerobic Checklist for Swimming

Pace Of Activity	Calories Burned		Aerobic Rating
	20 mins.	30 mins.	
Swimming (pleasure)	120	180	Medium
Swimming 1 lap in 1 min. 36 sec.*	160	240	High
Swimming 1 lap in 1 min. 15 sec.	220	330	High
Swimming 1 lap in 1 min.	250	375	High

*Note: 1 lap is one round trip in an Olympic-size pool or a total of 50 yards.

Drawbacks to Swimming

There are very few disadvantages to swimming as an aerobic activity. Those problems that do exist are easily remedied. One problem is that you need a good-sized pool for a workout. For most people, this means joining a club.

Another possible problem with swimming is the danger of ear, eye and sinus infections. Eye and sinus infections can be avoided with goggles and a nose clamp or a scuba mask. Ear infections can be avoided with earplugs.

If you are swimming in a public pool, the chlorine can do a number on your skin and hair. Good creams and conditioners help.

The last disadvantage of swimming is that it does require learning some skills, if you don't know how to swim. Most Y's offer swimming lessons.

Note from Joely

I was not an especially good swimmer when I first started. I hated putting my face into the water, which I attribute to my never having learned to breathe properly while swimming. I went through several months of straining to keep my head out of the water. Needless to say, I didn't make much progress. At about this time, we started taking scuba lessons. As part of the preliminary lessons, we had to practice using the scuba mask and snorkel in the pool. What a difference! I could breathe and I didn't have to twist my head back and forth. Now I won't even consider going swimming without my mask and snorkel.

If you want to get a scuba mask and snorkel, go to a good diving shop. They're the best people to help you get properly fitted. The cost of a good mask can run between $35 and $70, but for me it was well worth it. The kids really enjoy the masks, and they are now standard equipment for the beach.

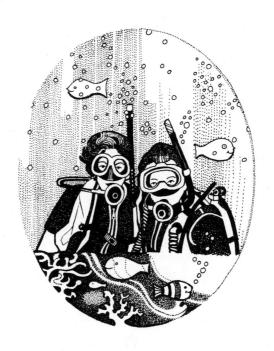

Your Personal Start-up Plan

We've included two plans, one for under 30 and one for over 30. If you're over 30 and have maintained step 12 of your start-up plan for a while, don't be afraid to upgrade to the under 30 chart. We did that after the first year of our program and during the second year we added running. Now we run and swim in the "under 30" program. The 3% formula works!

PERSONAL START-UP PLAN FOR SWIMMING
(Healthy, Under 30)

WEEKLY GOALS

Step	What To Do	Times Per Week	No. of Laps*	Time Per Lap	Flexi- bility‡ (Mins.)	Total Hrs:Mins. Per Wk.
1	swim	4	8	1.9 min.	20	2:21
2	swim	4	8	1.6 min.	20	2:11
3	swim	4	10	1.5 min.	20	2:20
4	swim	4	10	1.3 min.	20	2:12
5	swim	4	12	1.8 min.	20	2:46
6	swim	4	12	1.3 min.	20	2:22
7	swim	4	14	1.4 min.	20	2:38
8	swim	4	16	1.3 min.	20	2:43
9	swim	4	18	1.3 min.	20	2:54
10	swim	5	18	1.3 min.	20	3:37
11	swim	4	20	1.2 min.	20	2:56
12	swim	5	20	1.2 min.	20	3:40

*A lap is one round trip in an Olympic-size pool (50 yards or 150 feet).

‡See the next chapter for step-by- step directions for a flexibility program. We recommend a 20-minute flexibility program five days a week, so you'll be doing additional flexibility training on days when you do not do aerobic exercise.

PERSONAL START-UP PLAN FOR SWIMMING
(Healthy, Over 30)

WEEKLY GOALS

Step	What To Do	Times Per Week	No. of Laps*	Time Per Lap	Flexibility‡ (Mins.)	Total Hrs:Mins. Per Wk.
1	swim	4	6	2.0 min.	20	2:08
2	swim	4	6	1.6 min.	20	1:58
3	swim	4	8	1.6 min.	20	2:11
4	swim	4	8	1.5 min.	20	2:08
5	swim	4	10	1.4 min.	20	2:16
6	swim	4	10	1.3 min.	20	2:12
7	swim	4	12	1.3 min.	20	2:22
8	swim	4	14	1.4 min.	20	2:38
9	swim	4	16	1.4 min.	20	2:50
10	swim	4	18	1.2 min.	20	2:46
11	swim	5	18	1.2 min.	20	3:28
12	swim	5	20	1.2 min.	20	3:40

*A lap is one round trip in an Olympic-size pool (50 yards or 150 feet).

‡See the next chapter for step-by- step directions for a flexibility program. We recommend a 20-minute flexibility program five days a week, so you'll be doing additional flexibility training on days when you do not do aerobic exercise.

Walking

Walking is a natural, healthy activity. When you walk fast enough and far enough, you can derive the same benefits that you get from other aerobic activities.

Positive Checklist for Walking

* It can be done by almost everyone, regardless of age or condition.

* It requires no particular skill.

* There is a low risk of injury.

* It can be an individual or social activity.

* You can perform other activities while walking.

Aerobic Checklist for Walking

Pace Of Activity	Calories Burned 20 mins.	30 mins.	Aerobic Rating
Walking 1 mile in 30 min.	50	75	None
Walking 1 mile in 20 min.	80	120	Low. This is for people who can't exercise vigorously.
Walking 1 mile in 17 min.	100	150	Medium
Walking 1 mile in 15 min.	120-140	180-210	High
Walking 1 mile in 12 min.	160	240	High

Drawbacks to Walking

The basic drawback to walking is that it requires more personal time to get aerobic benefits than most people are willing to invest.

Your Personal Start-up Plan

There are two plans for walking, one for those under 30 and one for those over 30. At any time you can upgrade to running. For example, if you are over 30 and have completed and maintained step 12 in the over-30 start-up plan, you can easily go to a 14-minute mile without too much effort if your body tells you that it's okay!

A word of caution: If you have chosen walking as your primary aerobic activity because of some physical problem or on the advice of your physician, be very careful about upgrading to running. Don't do it without the professional advice of your physician. Swimming or biking may be better alternatives or complementary activities.

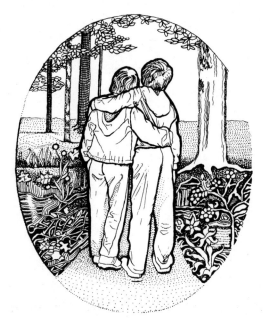

PERSONAL START-UP PLAN FOR WALKING
(Healthy, Under 30)

WEEKLY GOALS

Step	What To Do	Times Per Week	Miles	Minutes Per Mile	Flexi-bility* (Mins.)	Total Hrs:Mins. Per Wk.‡
1	walk	5	1.0	17	20	3:05
2	walk	3	2.0	17	20	2:42
3	walk	4	2.0	16	20	3:28
4	walk	5	2.0	15	20	4:10
5	walk	5	2.5	15	20	4:48
6	walk	5	2.5	14.5	20	4:41
7	walk	5	2.5	14	20	4:35
8	walk	5	3.0	15	20	5:25
9	walk	5	3.0	14.8	20	5:22
10	walk	5	3.0	14.5	20	5:18
11	walk	4	3.0	14	20	4:08
12	walk	5	3.0	14	20	5:10

*See the next chapter for step-by- step directions for a flexibility program. We recommend a 20-minute flexibility program five days a week, so you'll be doing additional flexibility training on days when you do not do aerobic exercise.

‡The 3% formula of five hours doesn't apply to walking.

PERSONAL START-UP PLAN FOR WALKING
(Healthy, Over 30)

WEEKLY GOALS

Step	What To Do	Times Per Week	Miles	Minutes Per Mile	Flexibility* (Mins.)	Total Hrs:Mins. Per Wk.‡
1	walk	5	1.0	18	20	3:10
2	walk	3	2.0	18	20	2:48
3	walk	3	2.0	17	20	2:42
4	walk	4	2.0	16	20	3:28
5	walk	5	2.0	15	20	4:10
6	walk	4	2.5	15.6	20	3:56
7	walk	5	2.5	15.2	20	4:50
8	walk	5	2.5	15	20	4:48
9	walk	5	3.0	15.5	20	5:33
10	walk	5	3.0	15	20	5:25
11	walk	4	3.0	14.5	20	4:14
12	walk	5	3.0	14.5	20	5:18

*See the next chapter for step-by- step directions for a flexibility program. We recommend a 20-minute flexibility program five days a week, so you'll be doing additional flexibility training on days when you do not do aerobic exercise.

‡The 3% formula of five hours doesn't apply to walking.

Biking

Do you remember your first bike? Dave got his first bike in the middle of the Second World War. You couldn't buy a new bike or car in those days. So...it was a used bike shared with his younger brother. Nevertheless, memories of those exciting days still provide the ambiance for today's biking activities.

Bikes are more exciting today than they were 30 or 40 years ago. You can get 5, 10, even 15 gears on a bike. If you like gadgets, there's an endless selection.

One of our friends took up biking in his mid-fifties as a way to control his blood pressure. Since he is an avid collector of gadgets, he has gradually upgraded the quality of his riding machine as his biking skills have improved. He currently has a $1200 bike that you can pick up with your little finger. For the more economical, you can get a halfway decent multi-speed bike for around $200 to $300.

Biking also can be linked to various social groups. The Appalachian Mountain Club, for example, sponsors various tours and trips. They can be a lot of fun for those in good shape!

Positive Checklist for Biking

* There is less strain on muscles and joints than in running or cross-country skiing.

* For most people, biking is fun! It brings back memories of happy childhood adventures and provides lots of fresh air!

* In many cases, you can bike rather than drive or take public transportation.

* Biking can be an individual or group activity.

* You can collect and tinker with different kinds of biking machines.

* There are numerous tours, clubs and social groups for cross-country trips and weekends.

The following aerobic checklist gives you an idea of how many calories can be burned while you bike.

Aerobic Checklist for Biking

Pace Of Activity	Calories Burned 20 mins.	30 mins.	Aerobic Rating
Biking 6 mph	80	120	Low. This is for people who cannot exercise vigorously.
Biking 10 mph	120	180	Medium
Biking 11 mph	140	210	Medium
Biking 12 mph	180	270	Medium
Biking 13 mph	220	330	High

Drawbacks to Biking

Some of the drawbacks to biking as a regular aerobic exercise include bad weather and careless motorists. You can avoid getting hit by a car by riding when there are very few cars on the roads or biking on special paths forbidden to cars. You should also wear protective headgear if you plan on doing a lot of biking. Stationary bikes help you to avoid many of the problems associated with biking outdoors. Just like regular bikes, stationary bikes come in different price ranges. You can buy stationary bikes that are controlled by computers. They allow you to select from a number of increasingly difficult levels that include warm-ups, hills, etc. You can also get a basic exercise bike for a more modest investment.

Your Personal Start-up Program

There are two programs, one for those under 30 and another for those over 30. The two programs end up at the same point, eight miles for each day at 15 mph (four-minute miles). If this is not strenuous enough for you, you can speed up a bit or add a mile to the run. Use your common sense and listen to your body. Unless you fall or get hit by a car, it's pretty hard to hurt yourself by pedaling.

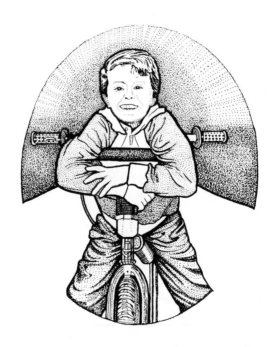

PERSONAL START-UP PLAN FOR BIKING
(Healthy, Under 30)

WEEKLY GOALS

Step	What To Do	Times Per Week	Miles	Mins. Per Mile	Miles Per Hour	Flexi-bility* (Mins.)	Total Hrs:Mins. Per Wk.
1	pedal	3	5	6	10	20	2:30
2	pedal	3	5	5	12	20	2:15
3	pedal	4	5	4	15	20	2:40
4	pedal	4	6	4.5	13	20	3:08
5	pedal	4	6	4	15	20	2:56
6	pedal	4	7	4.5	13	20	3:26
7	pedal	4	7	4	15	20	3:12
8	pedal	4	8	4.5	13	20	3:44
9	pedal	4	8	4.3	14	20	3:38
10	pedal	4	8	4	15	20	3:28

*See the next chapter for step-by-step directions for a flexibility program. We recommend a 20-minute flexibility program five days a week, so you'll be doing additional flexibility training on days when you do not do aerobic exercise.

PERSONAL START-UP PLAN FOR BIKING
(Healthy, Over 30)

WEEKLY GOALS

Step	What To Do	Times Per Week	Miles	Mins. Per Mile	Miles Per Hour	Flexi-bility* (Mins.)	Total Hrs:Mins. Per Wk.
1	pedal	3	4	6	10	20	2:12
2	pedal	3	4	5	12	20	2:00
3	pedal	4	5	6	10	20	3:20
4	pedal	4	5	5	12	20	3:00
5	pedal	4	5	4.5	13	20	2:50
6	pedal	4	6	4.3	14	20	3:03
7	pedal	4	6	4	15	20	2:56
8	pedal	4	7	4.5	13	20	3:26
9	pedal	4	7	4.3	14	20	3:20
10	pedal‡	4	7	4	15	20	3:12
11	pedal	4	8	4.2	14	20	3:34
12	pedal	4	8	4	15	20	3:28

*See the next chapter for step-by- step directions for a flexibility program. We recommend a 20-minute flexibility program five days a week, so you'll be doing additional flexibility training on days when you do not do aerobic exercise.

‡Acceptable aerobic fitness can be maintained here. We recommend going to step 12 and maintaining the pace.

Cross-Country Skiing

One solid hour of cross-country skiing is a perfect substitute for any primary aerobic program that you select. You don't need a chart to know how great a workout you're getting! In addition to using your legs, you use your upper body and arms to push with the poles.

Cross-country skiing is fun for all the family. It contains all of the social advantages of downhill skiing and is a lot less hazardous.

Positive Checklist For Cross-Country Skiing

* More aerobic benefits than running... more of your muscles are involved.

* Can be an individual, social and/or family activity.

* Organized groups sponsor weekends and other programs.

* Easier to learn than down-hill skiing.

* Can be a competitive sport, if you like.

* Designer clothes and colorful equipment are available.

Drawbacks to Cross-Country Skiing

Other than the need for special facilities, equipment, clothing, ideal weather conditions and the moderate risk of injury there is only one other drawback to cross-country skiing: it requires more skill than other aerobic activities. You'll probably want to take lessons.

CHAPTER TEN WORKSHEET

Long-term Goal(s) _____ Rewards _____

Exercise aerobically 20-minutes a day, 4 days per week.

Short-term Goals _____ Rewards _____

Make an appointment for a physical exam.

Reminder Notes: _____

See your physician for a checkup before starting.

Determine your exercise heart rate.

NOTES

CHAPTER ELEVEN

Maintaining Youthful Flexibility

Why Is Flexibility So Important?

Flexibility is a hallmark of youth. We're sure you can remember when you were younger and flexibility was something you took for granted. You could twist and turn your body in all sorts of ways without really thinking about it. What happened? What caused you to become stiff and sore? People are born flexible. Is it a sad fact of life that the flexibility disappears over time? Absolutely no! If you start young enough, you can maintain youthful flexibility throughout your life.

What about those of you who have already lost some flexibility...is it gone forever? Again, absolutely no! The wonderful thing about flexibility is that you can regain it **at any age.** Flexibility is synonymous with stretching. The more you stretch and the more parts of your body you stretch, the more flexible you become. We recommend a flexibility and stretching program that is the oldest known program in existence, Yoga. A major goal of this program is to break the vicious circle that begins when you become less active. This inactivity means that the

You can regain flexibility at any age.

169

spine becomes a little stiffer. As the spine becomes stiffer you often cut down even more on your activity which in turn allows the spine to become even stiffer, etc., etc., until you end up in a nursing home unable to take care of yourself (if you live that long.) **There is another way!**

Won't aerobics make me flexible? Why do I need a flexibility program *and* an aerobics program?

Remember that the goal of an aerobics program is to keep your heart and lungs healthy, not to increase or even maintain flexibility. In fact, most aerobic exercises lead to inflexibility of certain parts of the body. Swimming is an exception because it exercises the upper body as well as the lower, but even swimming doesn't have the overall benefits that can be derived from the program we recommend. It is a medical fact that muscles shorten and contract as your body moves. When a muscle is contracted, it cannot absorb blood. Since blood carries oxygen to the muscles, this means that the muscles are not getting as much oxygen as they could. The more oxygen your muscles can absorb, the healthier they are. Stretching lengthens muscles, which allows for improved blood flow. Poor circulation, on the other hand, is responsible for pain, which causes further contraction, which causes further pain, etc., etc. Again, a vicious circle.

When muscles are tight, your muscles do not get enough oxygen.

Joints are affected by muscles that are too tight. A joint that is surrounded by contracted muscles does not have the full range of motion that it was meant to have, and the body, being the amazing thing that it is, compensates by making some other joint do more work. This pulls the body out of alignment which further compounds your stiffness problems, etc., etc.

What are the differences between a flexibility program and regular exercise?

If you have ever done any kind of calisthenics, we're sure you will catch the similarity of these poses to typical exercises. It is only the most fleeting similarity, however, because yoga poses are far superior in their ability to improve flexibility and reduce tension. Calisthenics emphasizes quick jerking motions which snap the muscles. The major emphasis is on motion. In yoga, there is a negative emphasis on motion. They are called **poses** for a reason, and the reason is that yoga emphasizes holding muscles in a gentle stretch with a gentle release. Imagine a rubber band. In calisthenics, the goal is to pull the band out and snap it back quickly. In yoga, the goal is to stretch the rubber band very slowly, to hold it and then to release it gently. The muscles and spinal column are getting an excellent workout without the risk of injury inherent in calisthenics.

What is the Methuselah approach to flexibility?

The Methuselah approach uses Yoga, the oldest known science of self-development. It is aimed at providing everyone with the ability to solve their health problems, maintain physical fitness, obtain peace of mind and delay the aging process.

The Methuselah approach requires only 20 minutes a day five days a week for your flexibility program. That's less than one TV movie a week or five half-hour programs. Isn't your health worth that much to you?

WHAT CAN YOGA DO FOR ME?

Benefits of a Flexibility Training Program

PSYCHOLOGICAL BENEFITS

* Complete relaxation at will

* Relief of tension

* Relaxation of your nervous system

* Better sleep

* Quieter mind

* Improved self-concept

PHYSICAL BENEFITS

* Resilient muscles, taut skin

* Increased energy and vitality

* Increased suppleness and flexibility

* Improved complexion and a more youthful appearance

* Stronger and cleaner lungs

* Normal bowels and weight

* Trim body, improved circulation

What Are the Risks in a Personal Flexibility Program?

As far as we know, there are none! Unlike calisthenics, a yoga personal flexibility program involves gentle stretching movements and the holding of poses while concentrating on breathing and relaxation. When Dave taught yoga, he told his students, "If you hurt yourself in yoga, you are by definition not doing yoga!" **CAUTION: In order not to injure yourself, yoga flexibility and stretching exercises should be done slowly and gently. If you have any physical problems or injuries, get your physician's approval before beginning.**

Tell Me More About Yoga!

The science of Yoga has no temples, no creeds, no rites. Anyone from any religion (or no religion) can adopt it. It is a time-tested method with over 6000 years of experience in self-development programming!

The branch of Yoga that we are concerned with is called Hatha Yoga. It is the oldest known physical culture in the world. In recent years, western scientists and physicians have studied Hatha Yoga with modern equipment and techniques. The results of countless tests and experiments have increasingly shown that the practice of yoga does make profound physiological and psychological changes in human beings.

A Case Study

Seljarajan Yesudian, in his book *Yoga and Health*, recounts his personal story of how yoga transformed him from a sickly child into a healthy, vibrant boy. Although he was the son of a well-known and wealthy physician, he had had almost every major disease by the time he was fifteen – scarlet fever, dysentery, typhus, cholera and many other contagious diseases typical of a tropical climate such as India's. As a result, the boy was nothing but skin and bones with little energy and no strength. He tells of how he envied the boys in his school who could run and play while he could only look on wistfully from a corner of the school yard.

As is often the case with bright kids who are prevented from playing with friends, he turned to reading and found numerous books on Yoga philosophy and practice in his father's library. As a result of the enthusiasm these books inspired, he eventually found a teacher. According to his own report, he was a changed person within two months. At the end of a year his chest had increased four inches, his arms and legs had just about doubled in size, and he was never sick again.

If you could see the pictures of him demonstrating yoga poses in his book, you would certainly agree that he is in superb shape.

Some of you are probably scowling over this case study because you are saying to yourself, "Heaven forbid I should double the size of my legs! I need to lose weight, not gain it!" Joely's experience with yoga should be more encouraging for you.

Note from Joely

My first experience with yoga was about 13 years ago when I took a yoga course at a local YWCA. I enjoyed the course, although I was somewhat discouraged to find that I was not nearly as flexible as I assumed I would be. I had always been a fairly active child and was a cheerleader in high school, doing all the jumping and tumbling involved in that. It never occurred to me that I might be tightening up and losing the flexibility that I assumed would always be there, sort of as my God given gift. It was a rude awakening to discover that I couldn't do some of the "simple" bending and stretching positions as well as I thought I should be able to. The real killer was the leg stretch pose described later in this chapter. In this pose, you sit on the floor, bend forward, and stretch so that you rest your head on your knees. I could no more get my head anywhere near my knees than I could fly. I was lucky if I could bend down a third of the way, and I was only in my early twenties and considered myself in good shape. It added insult to injury when I noticed a woman in her fifties who was able to put her forehead flat to her knees as if she were hinged at the hips. (When I was 20, 50 was old. Ah, foolish youth!) I made a point of speaking to her during the class and she told me that she had been studying yoga for a couple of years. She assured me, however, that she had been in no better shape than I when she started (the nerve of her to notice!). During the time I spent in that course, I also noticed that while I was doing yoga I was satisfied with eating less than I usually did.

At that time in my life I was a classic example of the spirit being willing but the flesh being weak. My motivation was also limited to finding an enjoyable form of exercise so I never did any research into what yoga could really do for me. As a result, I never followed through on the program.

About four years ago under David's influence I went back to yoga. At the same time, I changed my eating habits so that they more closely resembled the diets we describe in the chapter on nutrition. I cut down drastically on sugar, salt and white flour and completely cut out caffeine and red meat. Because I was trying to combat feelings of extreme tiredness in midmorning and midafternoon, I ate six times a day. I ate some fruit, nuts or yogurt around 10:30 and around 3:30 and had another small snack in the evening after dinner. David or our secretary would set an alarm to remind me that I was supposed to eat because it was getting to a point where I was rebelling against eating all the time. All I could think of was, "Oh, no, I have to eat again."

Within two months of practicing yoga and improving my diet, I experienced a great increase in vitality. Although I had not changed my diet to lose weight, my clothes began to fit differently. It seemed that I woke up one morning and had lost about 10 pounds without really trying. I attribute both the increased energy and the decreased weight to the interaction of the yoga and the diet. Without knowing it, I began to implement the Methuseleh Manual 3% formula. I can attest that it works! As a closing note, I am more flexible now than I was almost 15 years ago.

More about Hatha or Physical Yoga

The word "hatha" is made up of two Sanskrit roots, "ha" and "tha". "Ha" literally means "sun" but is interpreted to mean the flow of the breath through the right nostril. Similarly, "tha" means "moon" but is interpreted to mean the flow of the breath through the left nostril. Thus "hatha yoga" means "union of the two breaths".

Physical or hatha yoga places great emphasis on breath control as the fundamental way to gain control of the mind and body. The focus is on controlling the breath when stretching, moving or meditating. Breath control is a fundamental part of the flexibility program outlined in this chapter as well as the relaxation program discussed earlier in the book.

Although this is definitely not a book devoted to yoga, yoga is the oldest discipline to pursue longevity through physical fitness, proper nutrition, relaxation and stress reduction. Yogis view the body as the temple of the spirit. They also believe that it takes the mind much longer to mature than the body. Since mental and spiritual self-development takes a long time, the emphasis of yoga has been on keeping the body youthful so that the mind can fully mature. According to yoga philosophy, a person is not physically mature until age 35 and is not mentally mature until age 55.

The Four Goals of Your Flexibility Program

---

1. **BECOME MORE AGILE, FLEXIBLE AND TONED**

   A major goal of this program is to help you become more flexible, toned and agile. You have only to look at a person who has practiced this program for a few months to notice the difference it can make.

2. **LEARN TO RELAX AT WILL**

   This program will help you learn to relax your muscles completely at will, letting your body benefit from profound relaxation.

3. **HELP YOUR GLANDS AND INTERNAL ORGANS FUNCTION BETTER**

   This program will teach you how to stimulate your internal organs and glands in such a way that they function more efficiently. This includes helping your system to better eliminate the toxic substances that are the by-products of your digestive process.

4. **LEARN HOW TO CONTROL YOUR BREATHING FOR BETTER PERFORMANCE AND RELAXATION**

This program will help you learn how to control your breath as an aid to relaxation, respiration and physical performance.

In a flexibility program, what you think about and visualize is just as important as what you do when you move your body. The aim of this program is gaining mental control over your physical body. Part of the secret is breath control and part is the use of visualization techniques to enhance your performance. Modern sports medicine has recognized the value of this approach and many of the Olympic champions were trained to visualize their performance just prior to performing. They also were trained to use breath control as an aid to smooth physical functioning. The ultimate reality is that there is no true separation of mind and body. These are only abstractions that we use in order to study and explain human behavior and functioning.

The chart below contains both psychologically and physically-oriented tips on improving your performance and progress in a flexibility program.

**Eleven Ways To A Successful Flexibility Program:
A Psychological Approach**

---

1. **PAY ATTENTION TO ATMOSPHERE**

From a psychological point of view, atmosphere is critical to a successful flexibility program. Make it a point from the beginning to find a quiet private place. Comfort is also an important part of the atmosphere. It's helpful to have a padded rug under you. An exercise mat is also good. The standing positions can be done on a bare floor, but many of the other positions can be uncomfortable if done without any kind of cushion.

2. **SET FLEXIBILITY GOALS THAT ARE REASONABLE**

As we have discussed many time before, goals are important to successful performance of any task and to making permanent modifications in your behavior. In the case of your flexiblity program, it is important that your goals not only be measurable but that they be process oriented. If you establish unreasonable goals for yourself, you could easily pull a muscle. You would be stiff rather than flexible as result of the injury. Many people who have begun yoga programs in their fifties, sixties and seventies have made remarkable progress in rejuvenating themselves by using a short-term goal approach.

3. **HAVE LOTS OF SPACE**

In picking your location, make sure you have enough space so that you can stretch out on all four sides. Clear away any furniture that might be in the way.

4. **WEAR LOOSE CLOTHING**

For men, in private, bikini-type briefs are excellent and quite comfortable. Women may prefer to go without a bra if it tends to bind. When doing yoga in group sessions, running shorts and T-shirts or leotards are most often worn. Make sure your shorts have an elasticized waistband. You don't want anything cutting into you.

5. **MORE IS BETTER**

Your flexibility program should be done four to five times a week. Flexibility training is one case where a little is good and more is better. If you have the time, try doing it every day.

6. **COORDINATE WITH YOUR AEROBICS PROGRAM**

If you choose running or biking as your aerobic exercise, you should do your flexibility program after you exercise. Running in particular tightens your muscles; yoga stretches them out and releases the lactic acid buildup. Swimming, on the other hand, is not as tightening so you can alternate your aerobic and flexibility programs if you prefer. Of course, in order to do them both four to five times a week, there will be days when you will want to do them both. At any rate, psychologically, you will feel more relaxed if you follow your aerobic exercise with gentle stretching, breathing and visualization.

7. **DON'T DO FLEXIBILITY TRAINING ON A FULL STOMACH**

Wait at least two hours after eating or do it in the morning before breakfast. Many of the movements and postures are designed to massage internal organs. This can disturb your digestive process if your stomach is full.

8. **TREAT YOURSELF GENTLY**

The movements and postures in this flexibility program are not exercises. Understanding this basic concept is essential to successful performance. You should not be tired at the end of a flexibility session. In fact, you should be rested and relaxed. If you have sore muscles, you are not doing it correctly. **The idea is to stretch as far as you can without pain and then hold.** If you go too far or too quickly, you will hurt yourself.

9. **TAKE YOUR TIME**

Progress is never in a straight line. Some days you'll make more progress than others. Just take it easy, relax and let your body respond over time. One of the great things about this program is that you can start at any age and expect to make progress. There are any number of tremendous programs specifically for senior citizens that would put a person in his or her twenties to shame. All you have to do is look at some of the articles in *Yoga Journal* or some of the how-to books to see people in their seventies and eighties who have been doing yoga for only a few years standing on their heads or twisted like corkscrews and generally acting as if they had much younger bodies (which they do).

10. **DON'T GET COMPETITIVE**

Be noncompetitive with yourself and with others. If you treat this program competitively it won't work. The flexibility program is a time to "let go" as much as it is a time to control. You must listen to your body and your breathing and concentrate on them. Yoga is very much a here-and-now kind of thing. If you concentrate on achieving a goal, even if the goal is a perfect pose, you are in the future. In yoga, it is important to concentrate fully on what you are doing at any given moment. Do the best you can at what you are doing at the moment you are doing it. Don't worry about yesterday or tomorrow or another person.

11. **REWARD YOURSELF**

As we have said many times before, rewarding yourself is essential to the permanent modification of your behavior. Rewards do not have to be material ones. In fact, psychological rewards usually work best in the long run. One of the approaches that we have always used in yoga is to find a reward that requires us to apply our newly developed flexibility in a physical activity. Dave found great psychological satisfaction in going back to running after a 30 year layoff and not having a sore muscle from day one because he had been doing flexibility training for many years. Now that is one terrific psychological reward for a fifty year old man!

WARM-UP MOVEMENTS AND POSITIONS

This section shows you how to perform three important warm-up movements and positions. These should precede all other movements. They can also be done during the day in the office to relieve tension and can be performed prior to your aerobic activities.

CAUTION: In order not to injure yourself, yoga flexibility and streching exercises should be done slowly and gently. If you have any physical problems or injuries, get your physician's approval before beginning.

**Positive Checklist for Warm-up Movements and Positions
(Chest Expansion, Knees to Chest, Hands to Floor)**

---

* Help You Relax

* Help Get Rid of Flatulence

* Help Get Rid of Indigestion

* Relieve Tension in Chest

* Relieve Tension in Back

* Relieve Tension in Legs

Warm-up: Hands To Floor

The illustrations below guide you through the hands-to-floor warm-up. This movement is an excellent way to relax and prepare for either your flexibility program or your aerobic one.

How to Relax and Relieve Back and Leg Tension
(Hands-to-Floor Pose)

1. Stand straight with your hands by your side. Keeping your arms straight, slowly raise them in front of you and up towards the ceiling. When your arms are about shoulder high, begin to bend backwards as far as you can comfortably go. Remember, do not strain yourself. Go only as far as is comfortable.

Breathing: Inhale slowly as you bend backwards.

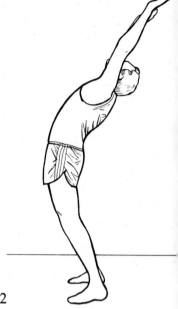

Visualization for Step 2

Concentrate on relaxing your back and neck. Create a visual picture of your leg muscles being stretched gently like rubber bands, slowly stretched to their limit. Think of your vertebrae as being gently pulled into alignment with lots of space around the disks. When you are touching the floor, think of your head as being free of the spinal column and hanging in space.

2. Keep your arms straight and bend forward at the waist until you can touch the floor or until you have gone as far as you can comfortably go. Try to keep your knees straight.

Breathing: Exhale as you bend forward and hold.

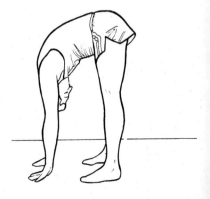

In this step don't just straighten up as you would in calisthenics. Think of your spinal column slowly rolling up like a roll-top desk, one vertebrae at a time, and the rubber bands in your legs being released ever so slowly and gently.

3.   **Slowly** curl up to a standing position.

Breathing: Inhale as you curl up.

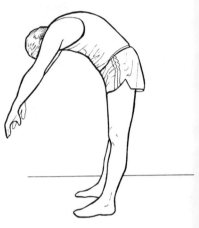

Additional Benefits of the Hand-to-Floor Pose

In addition to relieving back and leg tension, this pose has the following benefits:

* Massages the abdominal organs, helping with indigestion and constipation.

* Tones the liver, kidneys and pancreas.

* Improves menstrual disorders.

* Aids in weight loss.

* Trims the waist.

* Firms the legs.

* Invigorates the facial tissues.

Warm-up: Chest Expansion

This movement/posture is probably one of the best relaxation techniques we know. We do it as a way to unwind when working at the computer – about every thirty minutes when things are tense!

Keep your mind focused on relaxing the neck and lower back while you widen the chest.

How to Relax and Relieve Back, Chest and Leg Tension
(Chest Expansion)

As you do this movement, feel the tension between your shoulder blades as you bring your arms up to your chest.

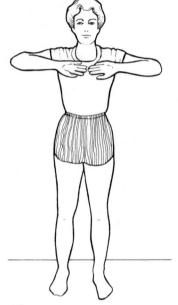

1.   Stand straight with your arms by your side. Bend your elbows and raise your arms so that the back of your hands touch your chest.

Breathing: Inhale.

Visualization for Step 2

As you bring your arms in back of you, feel the tension in your entire upper back, shoulders, chest and arms. Visualize the muscles across your chest and in your arms being gently stretched while the muscles in your back are being contracted.

2.   Bring your arms around in back of you and clasp your hands behind your back. Once your hands are locked, keep your elbows straight. Slowly bend backwards. Keep your arms as high as possible behind you.

Breathing: Hold your breath.

Visualization for Step 3

As you bend forward, relax the muscles in your neck and lead with your head. Imagine the rubber bands in your legs being stretched gently to their limit. Feel the tension in your shoulders and across your chest as your arms are stretched. Remember to release your neck from your shoulders and let it hang free when you are as far forward as you can go.

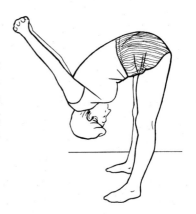

3. Slowly bend forward from the waist until your head is as close to your knees as you can move it. Keep your arms straight and your hands locked. Bring your hands over your head as far as you can. Hold the position for a count of 8.

Visualization for Step 4

Visualize your back as a rolltop desk rolling up one vertebrae at a time. As you roll up, feel the tension melting out of your neck, shoulders and chest. Feel the rubber bands in your legs releasing gently.

4. **Slowly** curl back up, keeping your hands locked and your arms straight. When you are standing, gently release your clasped hands.

Breathing: Exhale.

Additional Benefits of the
Chest-Expansion Pose

In addition to relieving back, chest and leg tension, this pose has the following benefits:

* Develops the bust or chest, which makes it an excellent companion for those people (particularly women) who choose running as their aerobic exercise.

* Firms the upper arms.

* Expands the lungs and stimulates the lung cells.

* Increases the blood flow to the brain. This helps to clear out the cobwebs and improves your mental functioning.

Don't be discouraged if you don't look like the picture the first time you try this pose. It is excellent for promoting flexibility of the spine, and you will improve a little every time you do it. Don't resort to the calisthenic bounce to increase your range. Remember, in yoga, slow and steady definitely wins the race.

Warm-up: Knees to Chin

This movement is an excellent warm-up technique for your aerobic program. It also will help you get rid of indigestion and flatulence. Do the right side first, then the left side and finish with both legs at the same time.

How To Relax and Relieve
Flatulence and Indigestion
(Knees to Chin)

Visualization Before Step 1

As you lie on the floor, take a deep breath and hold it for a moment. As you slowly exhale, feel the tension start to melt out of your body. Take another breath, release it slowly and feel your shoulders loosen and begin to sink into the floor. With your third breath, you can feel your spine and your leg muscles relax.

1.   Lie down on the floor and relax. Then bring your right knee to your chest. Use both hands to pull your knee down against your chest. Hold for a count of 8.

Breathing: Inhale as you bring your knee to your chest.

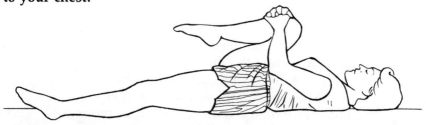

2.   Continue to hold your knee to your chest. Curl forward and bring your chin to your knee. Hold for a count of 8.

Breathing: Exhale.

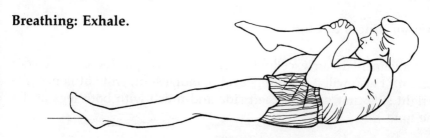

Imagine your back is a rolltop desk and you are rolling the vertebrae one by one to the floor. Feel the vertebrae being gently pulled into alignment as you roll back.

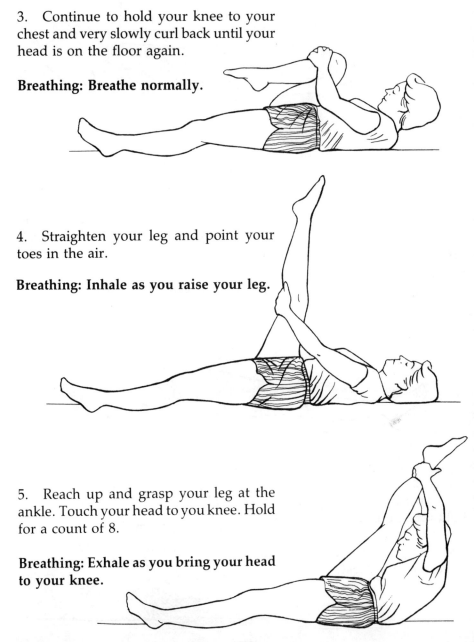

3.   Continue to hold your knee to your chest and very slowly curl back until your head is on the floor again.

Breathing: Breathe normally.

4.   Straighten your leg and point your toes in the air.

Breathing: Inhale as you raise your leg.

5.   Reach up and grasp your leg at the ankle. Touch your head to you knee. Hold for a count of 8.

Breathing: Exhale as you bring your head to your knee.

6. Keep your leg in the air while you slowly roll back to the floor.

Breathing: Breathe normally.

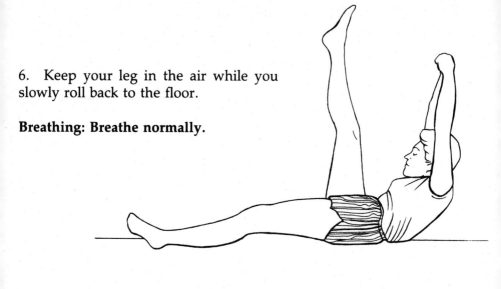

7. Place your palms against the floor for added support. Slowly lower the leg to the floor to a count of 8. (Lower the leg even more slowly if you can.) Keep the knee straight. Relax and then do the other leg.

Breathing: Breathe normally.

8. Clasp both knees to your chest and hold for a count of 8.

Breathing: Inhale as you bring your knees to your chest.

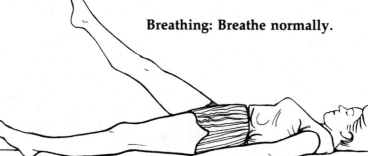

9. Bring your head to your knees and hold for a count of 8.

Breathing: Exhale as you raise your head.

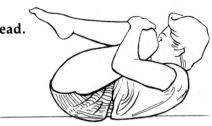

10. Very slowly roll back down to the floor.

Breathing: Breathe normally.

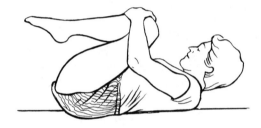

11. Place your palms against the floor. Point both legs straight up in the air.

Breathing: Breathe normally.

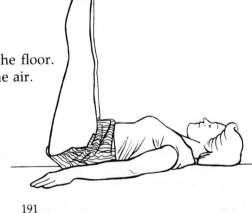

12. As slowly as you can, lower both legs to the floor. Relax.

Breathing: Breathe normally.

Additional Benefits of the Knees-to-Chin Pose

In addition to relieving flatulence and indigestion, the knees-to-chin pose has the following benefits:

* Develops ability to hold air in lungs, which makes it an excellent adjunct to aerobics. It is also a good pose for those with asthma.

* Improves flexibility of the hip joints.

* Strengthens abdominal muscles.

* Strengthens leg muscles.

* Massages internal organs.

STANDING MOVEMENTS AND POSTURES

These next series of movements and positions can be done between the chest expansion warm up and the knee to chin sets. The stomach lift should be done every day. The others can be omitted when you are pressed for time.

Positive Checklist for Standing Movements and Positions
(Eagle, Tree, Stomach Lift)

* Improve balance

* Strengthen ankles, legs

* Relieve tension in back

* Relieve tension in legs

* Promote good peristalsis

* Firm waistline

* Massage internal organs

Tree Pose

This is an excellent way to get rid of tension in the back and legs. It also helps you to improve your balance. Make sure that you focus your eyes on an object in the room in order to maintain your balance. If you don't, you will not be able to hold the pose. When you first start, you may have to stand next to a wall for support until you are into the position.

How To Improve Balance and Relieve Back and Leg Tension
(Tree Pose)

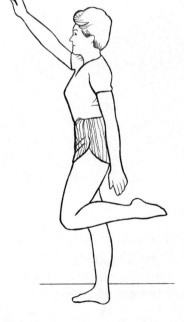

1. Stand straight and focus your eyes on an object in the room to help you maintain balance. Slowly raise your right arm. At the same time, bend your left leg at the knee and grab your ankle with your left hand.

Breathing: Inhale.

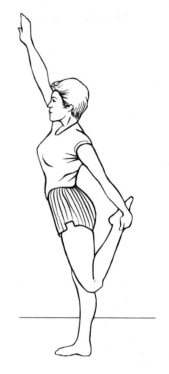

As you pull your leg back, bring the upper thigh as far back as you can. Feel the muscles stretch. Imagine the rubber band in the front of your upper leg being gently stretched to its limit.

2. Pull you heel **gently** towards your buttock. Point your right hand towards the ceiling. Hold for a count of 8.

Breathing: Exhale.

3. Slowly release your leg and lower it to the ground as you lower your hand. Repeat the same movements on the other side.

Breathing: Breathe normally.

Additional Benefits of the Tree Pose

In addition to relieving back and leg tension, the tree pose has the following benefits:

* Relieves tension in the shoulders.

* Develops poise and balance.

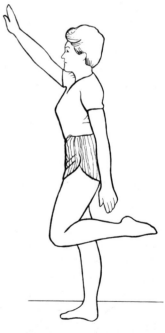

The tree pose is harder to do than it looks. You might want to do it against a wall so you can use your upraised hand to balance with if the need arises. The secret of balance is focusing your eyes on an object.

Eagle Pose

This is an excellent pose for improving your balance. It also helps to strengthen your ankles and legs. Make sure you keep your eyes focused on an object in the room in order to maintain balance. You may have to hold on to a chair to keep your balance at first.

How to Improve Your Balance, Strengthen Legs and Ankles
(Eagle Pose)

1. Stand straight with your hands at your side. Focus your eyes on an object in the room. Raise your arms out to the side to give yourself balance. Continue to focus on the object as you cross your right leg over your left leg.

Breathing: Breathe normally throughout this entire pose.

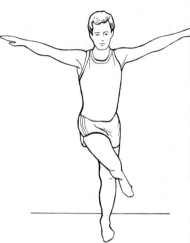

2. Hook your right foot behind the left ankle. Continue to focus on the object in order to maintain your balance.

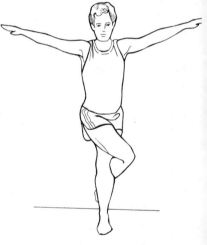

3. Cradle the elbow of your right arm inside the elbow of the left arm. Twist your left hand so that it faces out and then clasp your hands. Hold for 15 to 30 seconds. (Repeat steps 1, 2, 3 crossing left leg on right leg, etc.)

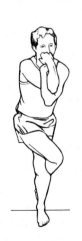

Additional Benefits of the Eagle Pose

In addition to improving balance and strengthening legs and ankles, the eagle pose has the following benefits:

* Increases the bust or chest. ·

* Improves flexibility of the knees.

* Strengthens calf muscles.

* Slims thighs.

* Tones up the muscles of the ankles, toes, knees, hips, shoulder joints, elbows, hands and fingers.

Stomach Lift and Stomach Roll

This movement stimulates the digestive tract, helps relieve constipation and massages many of your internal organs, including the liver, stomach, intestines and colon, and firms the waistline.

This should be performed three times every day. Experts in the science of yoga would rate this as one of the three most important movements. You may need a teacher to learn the "trick" of doing this, but it is well worth learning.

How to Firm Your Waistline, Relieve Constipation, Promote Peristalsis and Massage Your Internal Organs (Stomach Lift)

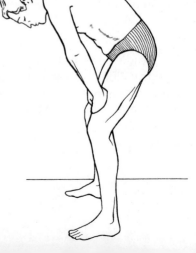

1. Stand in a semi-squat as shown. Place your hands on your thighs with the fingers facing inward. Blow all of the air out of your lungs by **pushing up with your stomach.**

Breathing: Exhale forcefully.

Don't just suck your stomach **in.** You want to suck it **in and up.** Imagine your belly button being sucked up into the rib cage as you suck your stomach in.

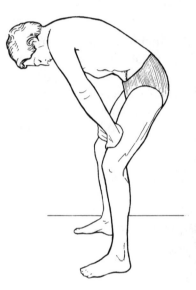

2. With your breath exhaled, suck your stomach in and up into your abdominal cavity, but don't let in any air.

3. "Flip" the abdomen in and out as many times as you can while keeping the breath exhaled. Don't just relax the muscles in order to let the abdomen go in and out; make sure you use the muscles to flip the abdomen.

Once you have mastered the stomach lift, begin to practice the stomach roll described next. Do the stomach roll right after the stomach lift while you are in the same position.

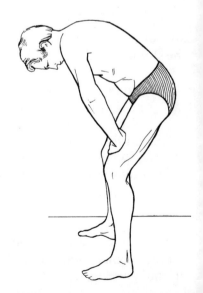

Stomach Roll

1. Maintain the semi-squat position described for the stomach roll. Increase the pressure of your hand on the right thigh and contract the muscles on the right side of your abdomen. Hold for a few seconds and release.

Breathing: Exhale forcefully.

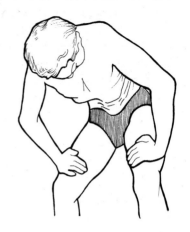

2. Increase the pressure of your hand on the left thigh and contract the muscles on the left side of your abdomen. Hold for a few seconds and release. Increase the tempo of contractions so that your stomach "rolls" from one side to the other.

Breathing: Keep breath exhaled.

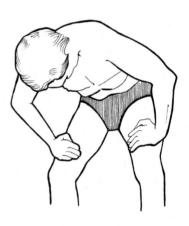

Additional Benefits of the Stomach Lift and Stomach Roll

In addition to firming your waistline, relieving constipation, promoting peristalsis and massaging your small intestine, liver, spleen, pancreas, gall bladder, stomach, and the reproductive glands and organs (as if that weren't enough), the stomach lift has the following benefits:

* Strengthens the back muscles that hold the abdominal muscles in place, helping to prevent backaches.

* Strengthens the abdominal wall, guarding against hernias.

* Firms abdominal muscles.

Note: Do these movements only on an empty stomach and preferably first thing in the morning.

HOW TO STAY YOUNG, HEALTHY AND SEXY:
THE BASIC POSITIONS

The movements and positions in this section form the foundation of the flexibility program and should be performed daily. The headstand is optional, depending on your physical condition.

INVERTED POSITIONS

This section shows you how to perform two very important positions – the headstand and the shoulder stand. If you ask anyone who has practiced the science of yoga for any period of time what three movements/positions, they would do if they could do no others, the answer would invariably be: (1) shoulder stand, (2) headstand and (3) stomach lift.

Positive Checklist for Inverted Positions
(Head and Shoulder Stands)

* Help delay aging.

* Help solve weight problems.

* Increase sex drive.

* Increase energy levels.

* Improve memory.

* Tone nervous system.

* Help digestive system.

* Stimulate endocrine system.

* Increase blood supply to brain.

* Increase blood supply to pineal gland.

* Increase blood supply to pituitary gland.

* Stimulate thyroid gland.

Shoulder Stand

The shoulder stand stimulates the endocrine glands and is believed to help delay aging. It is an excellent adjunct to a weight-control program because it stimulates the thyroid gland, which regulates the metabolism. Practitioners of the shoulder stand report increased sex drive and energy.

The objective is to invert the body and to trap blood in the thyroid gland area. If you are stiff or overweight you can prop yourself up on the wall. The object is to "get there" without hurting yourself no matter how long it takes.

How To Increase Energy, Sex Drive, Stay Young, Control Weight (Shoulder Stand)

1.   Lie down with your palms flat on the floor. Stiffen your legs and use your abdominal muscles to raise your legs so they are pointing at the ceiling.

Breathing: Breathe normally throughout this pose.

2.   Continue to bring your legs towards your head. Push down hard with your palms as you try to raise your waist and hips off the floor.

3.   When your hips are as far off the floor as you can get them, bring your hands up to your back to give yourself support.

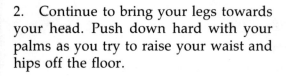
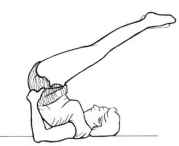

4. Slowly straighten your back so that your weight is primarily on your shoulders. Your arms should form a triangle of support with your back. Your chin should be pressed into the hollow of your throat. Hold for a count of 16. Work up to a count of 64. Advanced students hold for several minutes.

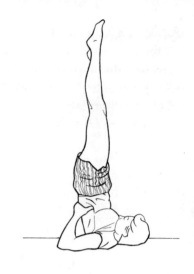

5. Coming out of the shoulder stand properly is as important as getting into it. Lower your legs towards your head and roll a few vertebrae onto the floor so that your weight is supported by your upper back and your arms.

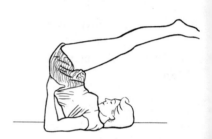

Visualization for Step 6

It is important that you do not come crashing down out of a shoulder stand, or any inverted position for that matter. Use your arms for support and imagine your back as the rolltop desk. **Slowly** roll your back onto the floor one vertebrae at a time.

6. When you feel balanced, place your palms flat against the floor and slowly roll down. Use your palms to steady yourself as you roll down.

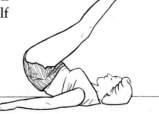

7.   When your back is flat on the floor, straighten your legs so that they point towards the ceiling. Slowly lower your legs to the floor. Then allow your body to go limp. Relax.

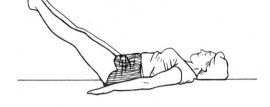

Note:
In the beginning you may want to "walk" up a wall in order to get yourself into the inverted position.

Additional Benefits of the Shoulder Stand

In addition to increasing your energy and your sex drive, helping to control your weight and helping you to stay young, the shoulder stand has the following benefits:

* Improves varicose veins, swollen feet and ankles.

* Diminishes hot flashes.

* Helps with displaced organs.

* Helpful for people with asthma because the increased blood supply stimulates the bronchioles and lungs.

Headstand

The headstand helps to increase the blood supply to the brain and the pineal and pituitary glands. It also helps to tone the nervous system. Practitioners and teachers report improved memory and digestion.

Known as the "king" of the yoga movements and positions, it is well worth your while to learn this one. Expect to spend several months learning it. As you will see in the instructions, you can master this pose in stages so you never need to go farther than you feel comfortable doing. Each of the intermediate stages puts you in an inverted position, however, so you derive tremendous benefits even though you have not completed the entire pose. You may want to have someone hold you in the beginning. You may also feel more comfortable with a teacher. Many people have learned this on their own and can attest to the physiological and mental changes it has induced.

There is also a new device available for doing the headstand without putting pressure directly on your neck. It looks like a padded stool except that a portion of the top can be removed, leaving an area that has been cut out for your neck. We certainly recommend this for those who have neck problems. You get the same effects but with the neck hanging free. Joely has found this method more relaxing than the traditional headstand although either will do the same thing for you physically.

CAUTION: If you have any blood pressure problems or injuries, get your physician's approval before beginning.

How To Improve Memory, Digestion, Tone Nervous System.
(Headstand)

1. Sit on your knees. Lean forward so that your forearms are on the floor. Interlace your fingers. Put your head between your hands with your forehead on the floor.

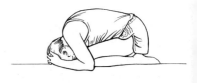

Breathing: Breathe normally throughout this pose.

If you are using an aid such as the one shown here, follow these directions:

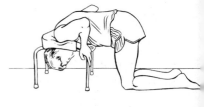

Sit on your knees. Lean forward and put your head into the cutout area so that you are resting on your shoulders. The rest of the steps are the same.

2. Raise your buttocks, lock your knees and "walk" towards your head as far as you can go.

When you first start practicing the headstand, you may want to stop at this step until you feel comfortable with it. It may also help to practice so that your back can straighten up against a wall.

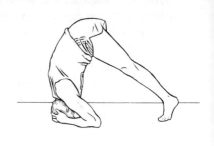

3. After you have walked as far as you can, use your toes to push off from the floor. Bend your knees as shown. Maintain your balance.

Again, you may want to go only as far as this step for a while until you feel comfortable with it.

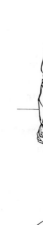

4. Slowly straighten your knees until your body is totally vertical. Hold for a count of 16. Work up to a count of 32. Advanced students hold this position for three minutes.

5. To let yourself down, bring your knees to your chest and balance yourself.

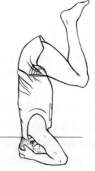

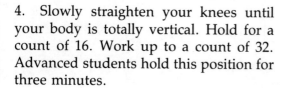

6. Slowly lower your legs until you are resting on your knees.

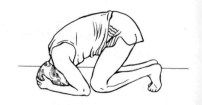

7. Lower your buttocks onto your heels. Put your arms behind you with the palms up. Relax in this position for a count of 32.

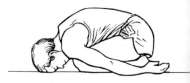

Additional Benefits of the Headstand

In addition to improving memory and digestion as well as toning the nervous system, the headstand has the following benefits:

* Enriches the pituitary and pineal glands, which in turn regulate the health of the thyroid, parathyroid, adrenals, and sex glands.

* Provides energy.

* Helps with sleeplessness, headaches, asthma, poor blood circulation, varicose veins.

* Excellent for women who have recently been through childbirth.

* Benefits eyes, teeth, hair, facial tissue.

CURVING THE SPINE FORWARD

This section shows you how to perform an important position: the plough. The plough helps keep your spine flexible while firming your stomach and normalizing your bowels.

Positive Checklist for Forward Spinal Curve
(Plough)

* Keeps spine flexible.

* Helps normalize bowels

* Helps firm stomach.

* Improves circulation.

* Helps you sleep better.

* Helps you relax.

The Plough

Initially, you may want to practice the plough by propping your feet against the wall and "walking" up the wall in order to get into the inverted position. After you have mastered the plough as described here, you can enter this pose directly from the shoulder stand.

How To Keep Spine Flexible, Normalize Bowels, Tighten Stomach
(Plough)

Preliminary Notes

Do this position with the aid of a chair or couch. Place the chair so that it is an arms's length above your head when you lie on the floor. Once you have mastered the position as described here, you can take away the chair and bring your feet to the floor beyond your head.

1. Lie on the floor with your palms down. Stiffen your legs and use your abdominal muscles to raise your legs so that they are pointing at the ceiling.

Breathing: Breathe normally throughout this pose.

2. Continue to bring your legs towards your head. Push down hard with your palms as you try to raise your waist and hips off the floor.

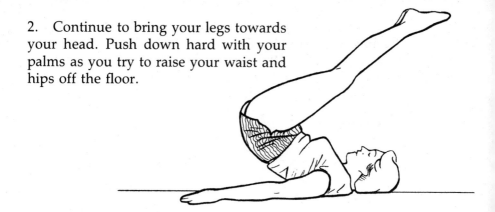

3. Put your hands against your back to help push yourself up. Bring your legs over your head and down to the chair. Do not bend the knees. If you can, take your hands away from your back and place your palms flat against the floor. Hold for a count of 16. Build up to a count of 64.

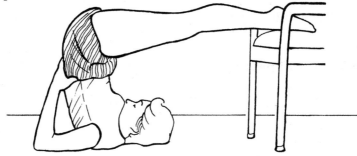

Advanced students can try the classic plough and bring their feet to the floor.

Visualization for Step 4

To come out of the plough, imagine the rolltop desk and **slowly** roll your back onto the floor one vertebrae at a time.

4. The trick to coming out of the plough is to roll your back to the floor first. Your legs will follow automatically. Use your palms to steady yourself as you roll down. When your back is on the floor, slowly lower your legs to the floor.

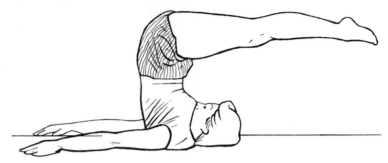

Additional Benefits of the Plough

In addition to keeping the spine flexible, normalizing the bowels and tightening the stomach, the plough has the following benefits:

* Reduces fatigue and exhaustion.

* Rejuvenates the sex glands, pancreas, liver, spleen, kidneys, as well as the suprarenal glands.

* Alleviates headaches.

* Good for people with diabetes because of the stimulation of the pancreas.

CURVING THE SPINE BACKWARDS

The section shows you how to perform two very important movements: the cobra and the bow. These movements are designed to help you keep your spine flexible and stimulate your internal organs and glands.

Positive Checklist for Backward Spinal Curves
(Cobra, Bow)

* Stimulate sex glands

* Keep spine flexible

* Stimulate internal organs

* Stimulate adrenals

* Prevent constipation

* Strengthen the back

* Tighten stomach, back muscles

* Tone buttocks, arms, legs

* Improve circulation

* Get rid of stomach gas

* Correct spinal curvatures

Cobra

The cobra stimulates the adrenals, abdominal organs and the sex glands. Practitioners and teachers report that it helps prevent constipation and strengthens the back.

One of the tricks to this movement is to roll the eyes slowly up and back as you perform. Visualize yourself looking up and over the top of your head.

How To Increase Sexual Energy and Keep The Spine Flexible
(The Cobra)

1. Lie flat on your stomach with your head turned to one side. Put your hands at shoulder level with the fingers pointing inward. Relax and then put your forehead on the floor.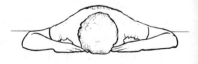

2. Begin to roll your eyes upward and at the same time lift your head and upper body off the floor.

Breathing: Inhale as you raise off the floor.

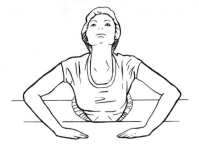

3. Arch your head and upper back towards your heels. Hold for a count of 8. Work up to a count of 16.

Breathing: Hold your breath.

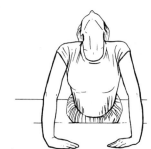

4. Slowly return to starting position. Allow your eyes to return to a normal position as you lower your upper body. Relax with cheek on floor.

Breathing: Exhale.

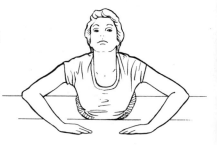

Additional Benefits of the Cobra

In addition to increasing sexual energy and keeping the spine flexible, the cobra has the following benefits:

* Stimulates the pancreas, liver and other organs of the digestive system.

* One of the best poses for alleviating constipation, indigestion, dysentery, flatulence, stomachaches, and other abdominal disorders. You may very well find yourself "burping" as you finish this pose.

* Excellent pose for increasing lung capacity and breath control.

* Strengthens heart and lungs.

* Stimulates adrenal glands.

* Stimulates the chest, shoulders, neck and face.

* Firms the bust.

The Bow

The bow helps to develop your chest and back. It improves posture and can help correct spinal curvatures. Practitioners and teachers report that it helps alleviate stomach gas and stimulates circulation. This is a powerful stretch; be sure to come out of it slowly.

How To Improve Posture, Spinal Curves, Alleviate Stomach Gas (The Bow)

1. Lie on your stomach with your chin on the floor. Bend one knee and reach back and grab the foot. Do the same with the other foot. Hold both feet as shown.

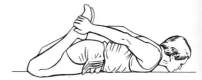

Breathing: Breathe normally.

2. Slowly raise your head and upper body off the floor. Next pull knees up from the floor in a steady motion. Hold for a count of 8.

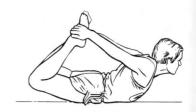

Breathing: Inhale.

3. Slowly lower your trunk and legs to the floor but don't let go of your legs until your trunk is all the way down. Slowly release your legs. Relax.

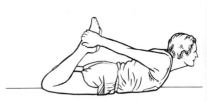

Breathing: Exhale.

Additional Benefits of the Bow

In addition to improving posture and spinal curves and alleviating stomach gas, the bow has the following benefits:

* Firms the bust, stomach, and thighs.

* Helps to regulate the functioning of the pancreas, which makes it an excellent pose for diabetics.

* Activates the adrenal, thyroid, parathyroid, pituitary, and sex glands.

* Improves flexibility of the shoulders, elbows, hips, knees and ankles.

LEG STRETCHES AND PULLS

This section shows you how to perform leg stretches and alternate leg pulls. These movements/positions are very good for keeping your spine flexible. They are also good for runners to perform after running.

Positive Checklist for Leg Stretches & Leg Pulls

* Help keep spine flexible

* Help correct constipation

* Tone stomach

* Tone back and legs

* Tone thighs

* Stretch legs and feet

* Strengthen back

* Get rid of stomach and thigh flab

Alternate Leg Pulls

Alternate leg pulls stretch your legs and feet. They are very good for runners, swimmers and cyclists. They help to get rid of stomach and thigh flab and strengthen the back.

How To Get Rid of Stomach and Thigh Flab and Strengthen Your Back (Alternate Leg Pulls)

1. Sit on the floor and place your right foot on the inside of your left thigh as close to the crotch as you can. Raise your arms above your head and bend backwards.

Breathing: Inhale.

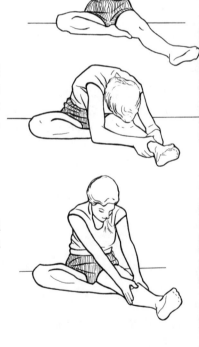

2. Twist towards your left leg and bend forward. Grab your left ankle with both hands. Lower your elbows to the floor and gently pull your head to your knee. Hold for a count of 8.

Breathing: Hold.

3. Slowly release your ankle and curl back up to a sitting position. Repeat with the other leg.

Breathing: Exhale.

Additional Benefits of Alternate Leg Pulls

In addition to getting rid of stomach and thigh flab and strengthening your back, alternate leg pulls have the following benefits:

* Massage abdominal organs.

* Slim the waistline.

* Stretch leg muscles and Achilles tendons, which makes these stretches an excellent adjunct to running and biking.

Leg Stretches

Leg stretches help to keep the spine flexible. They tone the back, legs and stomach. Practitioners and teachers report that they help correct constipation.

How To Tone Back, Legs and Stomach and Keep Spine Flexible (Leg Stretches)

Visualization for Step 1

The purpose of bending backwards is to give the spine maximum stretch in preparation for the next step. Imagine your spine being stretched gently to its maximum length with lots of space between the vertebrae.

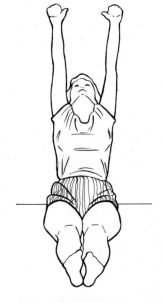

1. Sit on the floor with your legs together. Raise your arms above your head and bend backwards.

Breathing: Inhale.

Although the directions in Step 2 tell you to grab your ankles, you may not be able to reach them until you develop more flexibility. Grab hold of your legs **anywhere** you can reach, even if it is only your knees. We guarantee that if you keep practicing this pose, you will eventually be able to reach your ankles. As you pull your head towards your knees, imagine the rubber band in your spinal column stretching gently to its maximum length. In your mind's eye, see the spaces between the vertebrae expanding and the vertebrae themselves being pulled gently into alignment.

2. Bend forward and grab your ankles. Lower your elbows to the floor and slowly pull your head to your knees. Hold for a count of 8.

Breathing: Hold.

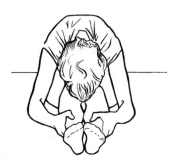

3. Release your ankles and slowly curl back up to a sitting position.

Breathing: Exhale.

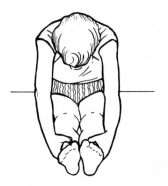

Additional Benefits of Leg Stretches

In addition to keeping the spine flexible and toning the back, legs and spine, the leg stretches have the following benefits:

* Massage abdominal organs.

* Slim the waistline.

* Stretch leg muscles and Achilles tendons, which make these stretches an excellent adjunct to running or biking.

KNEELING POSITIONS

This section shows you how to perform the classic kneeling positions, the diamond and child poses. Both poses are relatively easy to master and help you relax.

Positive Checklist for Kneeling Positions
(Diamond and Child Poses)

* Help you relax

* Strengthen knees

* Strengthen ankles, insteps

How to Kneel Relaxed:
The Diamond and Child Positions

Both positions are noted for helping you relax. The diamond pose helps to strengthen your ankles, knees and insteps. Practitioners and teachers report that it helps correct rheumatism.

Diamond Pose

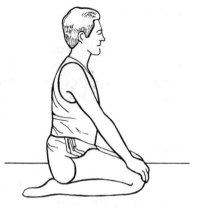

1. Sit on your heels, with back straight. Put your hands on your knees. Close your eyes and concentrate on filling your body with energy.

Breathing: Breathe in and out very slowly and rhythmically.

Note: The diamond pose can be adapted to improve hemorrhoids and tone up the vaginal muscles in women. When you are in the diamond pose as described above, inhale, exhale and tighten the muscles of the anus (and, for women, the vagina), drawing them up into the body. Hold for a few seconds and relax. Repeat.

Additional Benefits of the Diamond Pose

In addition to strengthening knees, ankles and insteps and helping you to relax, the diamond pose has the following benefits when practiced with the anal and vaginal contractions:

* Stimulates the reproductive system.

* Improves hemorrhoids.

* Improves prolapsed uterus in women.

* Improves enlarged prostate gland in men.

Child Pose

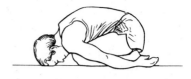

1. Sit on your heels. Lean forward and put your forehead on the floor. Put your arms at your sides with the palms facing up.

Breathing: Breathe in and out slowly.

Additional Benefits of the Child Pose

In addition to helping you relax and strengthening your knees, ankles and in-steps, the child pose has the following benefits:

* Relaxes the spine.

* Sends blood to the face and head.

* Tones the solar plexus.

GETTING STARTED

In a flexibility program such as the one we have just described, it is important to do the exercises in an order that allows for complementary flexing of the spine. In other words, you want to follow a pose that flexes the spine forward with one that flexes the spine in the opposite direction. Although the poses were presented in categories, you should practice them in the following order:

1. Hands to Floor, page 182.
You can do a second hands-to-floor pose, and as you roll up into a standing position, stop at the point where you can bend your knees and assume

the starting position of the stomach lift.

2. Stomach Lift and Stomach Roll page 196.

3. Chest Expansion, page 184.

4. Tree, page 193.

5. Eagle, page 194.

6. Knees to Chin, page 187.

7. Shoulder Stand, page 200.
   When you have held the fully inverted position with your feet straight in the air for as long as you can, go right into the plough by bringing your feet over your head.

8. Plough, page 206.

9. Cobra, page 209.

10. Bow, page 211.

11. Alternate Leg Pulls, page 213.
    When you finish with the alternate leg pulls, you can go right into the leg stretches.

12. Leg Stretches, page 214.

13. Diamond Pose, page 216.

14. Child Pose, page 218.

15. Headstand, page 202.
    You should be completely warmed up before you attempt the headstand. Follow the headstand with another child pose to relax.

KEEPING TO A 20-MINUTE PROGRAM

The entire program as outlined above will probably take 30 minutes. In order to keep to the 20 minutes we recommend as the minimum time to be allotted to a flexibility program, alternate the Group A and Group B poses, doing one or the other each day.

Personal Flexibility Program

Posture/ Movement	Page	Group A	Group B
1. Hands to Floor	182	x	x
2. Stomach Lift / Rolls	196	x	x
3. Chest Expansion	184	x	x
4. Tree	193	x	
5. Eagle	194		x
6. Knees to Chin	187	x	
7. Shoulder Stand	200	x	x
8. Plough	206		x
9. Cobra	209	x	
10. Bow	211		x
11. Alternate Leg Pulls	213	x	
12. Leg Stretches	214		x
13. Diamond Pose	216	x	
14. Child Pose	218		x
15. Headstand	202	x	x

CHAPTER ELEVEN WORKSHEET

Long-term Goal(s)   Rewards

_____

_____

_____

_____

Short-term Goals   Rewards

_____

_____

_____

_____

_____

_____

_____

_____

_____

_____

_____

_____

Make appointment with physician _____

_____

_____

_____

Reminder Notes:

_____

_____

_____

NOTES

SECTION FOUR

The Psychology
Of Controlling
Your
Body Chemistry

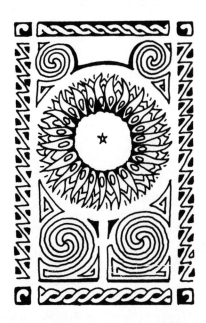

CHAPTER TWELVE
Long-Life Nutrition

In this chapter you will learn about the typical American diet and its effect on your health and the relationship of diet to various diseases. Also, you will learn about several basic nutritional programs which have been shown to reduce the risk of major diseases and therefore are considered long-life promoting. In addition, this chapter also provides you with a basic list of long-life foods and a step-by-step approach to making the transition from a short-life diet to a long-life nutrition program.

The Psychology of Food

How many times have you gone on a diet to lose weight? How many times have you been successful? How many times have you gained it all back? Unless you are very different from most Americans, you have been the "I'm going to lose five pounds" route at least once! And the chances are that you gained it all back. Right? Why? It's because:

"Diet" Is A Dirty Word!

That's right, "diet" is a dirty word. The word "diet" implies deprivation, even starvation, to many people. That's why poor eating habits are among the most difficult habits to modify. The word "diet" is an emotional word that often elicits feelings of guilt, resentment and frustration. There is also a part of you that associates a whole bunch of words, smells, and sounds, as well as social and sensual pleasures with eating. These are learned, but emotionally loaded, behaviors.

The development of emotional feelings about food and the need for oral gratification through food began the moment you were born. Food represents feelings of love, security, trust, sensory pleasure and gratification. When you are deprived of these associations, you feel it at an emotional level! As you grew up, this emotional attachment to food was constantly reinforced by your parents, peers and other significant adults. If you're like most of us, you were rewarded for good behavior with food and punished for bad behavior by withdrawal of food.

In addition, you associate food and the rituals of food with social functions and, oftentimes, religion. The food customs that you learned from society and religion took on emotional overtones also. For example, olives and caviar are considered "sophisticated" adult foods. Peanut butter and jelly brings back pleasant memories of growing up, and "quiet little dinners for two" are associated with sex. (Remember the movie *Tom Jones*?) Certain foods are said to have magical properties, and in some religious and cultural groups, some foods are considered taboo. A healthy steak and potatoes meal is considered very masculine, while a cucumber sandwich is considered appropriate for a ladies' garden party.

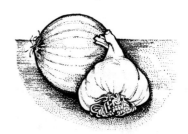

The point we are making here is that modifying your eating patterns is not going to be easy because it involves your feelings of love, security, social status, culture, trust and other powerful emotions. Fortunately, since eating habits are learned behavior, they can be modified by the same techniques you use to modify any learned behavior. In terms of food, the process involves learning the following things:

Ten Things To Learn About Eating Healthy

Source	Learning Tasks
Chapter 12	1. Acquire an understanding of the problems with the typical American diet.
	2. Learn about the relationship between diet, disease and stress.
	3. Learn about long-life diets that have been shown scientifically to decrease the risk of major diseases.
	4. Learn about food groups and specific foods that have been scientifically found to promote health and long life.
	5. Learn the criteria for selecting food that will help you stay young, healthy and sexy.
	6. Learn how to shop so that the food you eat contains only nutritious ingredients.
Chapter 13	7. Learn how to modify your nutritional program so that you can stick with it.
Chapter 14, 15	8. Learn what research says about specific vitamins and minerals, including deficiency symptoms.

Source	Learning Tasks
Chapter 16	9. Learn what research says about the therapeutic uses of supplements and using supplements to protect yourself from environmental poisons.
Chapter 17	10. Learn about methods of internal cleansing that claim to rid your body of toxins.

The American Diet

Regardless of where you live and what foods you eat, your diet will consist of simple and complex carbohydrates, protein, fat, vitamins, minerals, water, fiber and other nonnutritional elements. Depending on what you put in your mouth, the proportions of these elements will vary. For example, if you eat butter all by itself, you are eating almost pure fat. If you eat a spoonful of white sugar, you are eating a simple carbohydrate with little or no nutritional value. If you eat 100% stone-ground whole-wheat bread, you are getting almost all of the components on our list above.

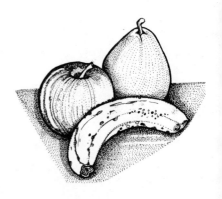

There are two issues in learning how to eat healthy foods: (1) How much of these various foods do I eat? and (2) What proportion of my total food intake should be made up of each of these ingredients? Fortunately, in recent years there has been increased scientific interest in nutrition and its effect on disease and longevity. Study after study shows that the typical American diet is unhealthy. Let's take a look at why your eating habits may be detrimental to your health.

Two Average-Life-Span Diets

Diet*	Major Elements‡
1. **TYPICAL, UNHEALTHY AMERICAN DIET**	**Too Much Fat:** The typical American diet consists of 40 to 45% fat. Diets this high in fat have been shown to cause cancer, diabetes and heart disease.

Too Much Protein: Actual daily protein requirements are around 5 to 10% of daily caloric intake. Excess protein overworks the kidneys, produces toxic residues and excess uric acid in the tissues and increases the urinary excretion of calcium.

Too Much Sugar: Most Americans get 25% of their daily calories from refined sugar. These are empty calories since sugar is so highly refined that all the nutrients and fiber have been removed. Regardless of its source, sugar is bad for you. It puts stress on your pancreas, raises the level of fat in your blood, can lead to hypoglycemia and contributes to the development of arteriosclerosis.

Not Enough Complex Carbohydrates: And too much salt, caffeine, alcohol and tobacco. Americans get only about 20% of their calories from complex carbohydrates. In contrast, people who live long and have a low risk of heart disease, cancer, etc., get somewhere around 75 to 80% of their calories from complex carbohydrates. When Americans do eat complex carbohydrates, they often eat highly refined and processed versions, such as polished white rice, that have lost a lot of valuable nutrients.

2. **U.S. SENATE NUTRITION COMMITTEE'S DIET RECOMMENDATIONS**

30% Fat: Thirty percent of your calories in fat is three times what you need.

12% Protein: Increasingly, research is showing that we need less, not more, protein. This is a step in the right direction, but there's still a long way to go.

15% Sugar: There is no scientific evidence to show that refined sugar is a nutritional requirement for anyone! In fact, all the evidence points to it as a serious addiction of many Americans, and one which leads to serious diseases.

43% Complex Carbohydrates: While this recommendation is in the right direction, Americans need to almost double this amount if they are to increase their chances of living longer and healthier lives and reducing the risk of heart disease, diabetes and cancer.

*The word "diet" is used to mean total nutritional intake. It does not mean a weight-loss program.

‡Nutrition is an extremely complex field. We are not nutritionists. In this chapter we are highlighting research findings in nutrition and health, our own experiences, and discussions with professionals in the field.

What About Diet and Disease?

Do you remember your history-book stories of scurvy and how it plagued the

British navy? When it was discovered that all they needed to prevent this from happening was fresh fruit and vegetables, the navy began to put citrus fruits in the galleys. This is how British sailors came to be known as "Limeys."

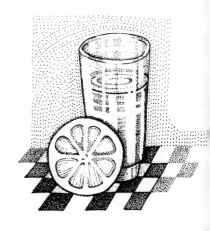

This classic story underscores how important good nutrition is to health and how poor nutrition can lead to disease and death. This next chart outlines the hard facts about the major dietary problems with the average American diet and why it has led to sharp increases in heart disease, gout, cancer, arthritis, hypoglycemia and diabetes.

Six Disease-Related Dietary Habits

Diet	What It Does To You
1. **HIGH-SALT DIET**	Salt makes your body retain fluids. It causes high blood pressure and is linked to kidney malfunction, breathing problems, obesity, stress-anxiety symptoms and may pave the way to arthritic conditions by causing bone degeneration. The fact is that you do not need to add salt to your food because it is present in its natural form in most foods.
2. **REFINED-SUGAR DIET**	Too much refined sugar can lead to hypoglycemia, or low blood sugar, by causing the pancreas to overreact and put out too much insulin. When a diet that is heavily laden with refined sugar is combined with a diet high in fat, it can lead to diabetes.
3. **DIET HIGH IN FOOD ADDITIVES**	Numerous additives such as nitrites, dyes and artificial sweeteners have been found to cause cancer in laboratory animals. While the use of additives and preservatives is still controversial, the evidence con-

Diet	What It Does To You
	tinues to mount that it may be safer to avoid foods which contain them.
4. **DIET HIGH IN REFINED FOODS**	Refined foods such as white flour, white rice and refined sugars have been linked to cancer when combined with a high-fat diet. They are nutritionally deficient, low in fiber and may contain additives.
5. **HIGH-FAT, LOW-FIBER DIET**	The high-fat, low-fiber diets of the modern industrialized world are all associated with an increase in heart disease and cancer.
6. **HIGH-PROTEIN DIET**	A diet high in protein can lead to an accumulation of toxic substances in the body, depletion of the vitamins and minerals in the body and higher levels of blood cholesterol, which can block your arteries. In addition, there is the risk of kidney and colon problems.

What About Diet and Stress?

Not only can a poor diet lead to serious diseases, the ingestion of certain substances can trigger your stress mechanisms. Chronic stimulation of your innate "fight or flight" response can also lead to disease.

Five Stress Producing Substances

Substance	What It Does To You
1. **CAFFEINE**	Recent studies show that two cups of coffee decrease blood flow to the brain. Caffeine stimulates your heart, breathing and

Substance	What It Does To You
	nervous system and triggers the entire stress-response mechanism. Caffeine is particularly hard on the liver, pancreas and other parts of the "fight or flight" mechanism. It drives water-soluble vitamins out of your system and lowers your resistance.
2. **SUGAR**	White refined sugar (sucrose) is commonly labeled by nutritionists as an "empty calorie" food because it does not contain one single nutrient. Like caffeine, it triggers the stress response, with the same fallout. Your body has no known physiological need for sugar. In addition, there is research evidence that shows that it may be a major cause of obesity. Sugar is also a major factor in tooth decay and diabetes. There is also some evidence that it may be linked to heart disease.
3. **DRUGS**	Our society pops pills like the ancients ate grapes. These drugs also stimulate the stress-response mechanism. Drugs deplete your body of essential vitamins and minerals as well as causing addiction.
4. **ALCOHOL**	Alcohol destroys the liver, taxes the kidneys and pancreas, and puts a strain on the body's detoxification system. There is some evidence that immoderate consumption is linked to cancers of the head and neck. Even in moderation, alcohol uses up many essential vitamins and minerals.
5. **TOBACCO**	In addition to depleting your body of vital nutrients, tobacco is linked to cancer of the lungs, mouth and throat.

What Diets Are Good For Me?

Long-lived modern-day Methuselahs eat a diet comprised primarily of complex carbohydrates, with very little meat, fat, processed or refined foods. The chart below describes three approaches to nutrition. Clinical and scientific research evidence shows that people on these diets have fewer major diseases.

Three Long-Life Nutritional Approaches

Diet	Features
1. **MACROBIOTICS**	**Basics:** The macrobiotic diet as described in most of the literature consists of 50% whole grains, 25% cooked vegetables, and 10% beans. The remaining 15% is composed of sea vegetables, condiments, fresh fruits and natural sweeteners.
	Restrictions/Special Features: Macrobiotics does not allow vegetables from the nightshade family, specifically potatoes, eggplant and tomatoes. It focuses on eating locally grown and seasonal food. Artificial ingredients, refined food and sugars, red meat and dairy products are excluded.
	History: It is based on the diet of Japanese monks who have a history of long life and good health. Although macrobiotic approaches are not always considered "scientific," there is some research data and clinical evidence based on one-shot case studies that support the claims that they can be effective in maintaining good health for many people.

2. **PRITIKIN**

Basics: The Pritikin diet is designed to give you a daily intake of 10% fat, 10% protein and 80% complex carbohydrates.

Restrictions/Special Features: All vegetables and fruits are eaten except olives and avocados, both of which have too much fat. A small amount of lean red meat is allowed. Low-oil fish and poultry without skin are also permitted within the 10% fat allowance. No distinction is made between animal and vegetable fat. Skim milk and low-fat cheeses are also permitted. Alcohol, smoking, caffeine, and all refined sugars are forbidden.

History: The track record of Pritikin's Longevity Center in the use of this diet to treat such diseases as diabetes, high blood pressure, gout, heart disease, arthritis and circulatory ailments is most impressive. More than 50% of those with adult-onset diabetes leave the clinic insulin-free, and 85% of those with high blood pressure leave with lower blood pressure and off medication. The record is similar with gout. Seventy percent leave the clinic off medication and symptom-free. Cholesterol levels drop 25% on the average.

3. **VEGETARIAN**

Basics: Diets vary according to philosophy. The one thing that the various kinds of vegetarians share in common is that they do not eat the flesh of animals or fish.

Restrictions/Special Features: There are several varieties of vegetarians:

Vegans are strict vegetarians who will eat only plant food (fruits, vegetables and grains).

Lacto-ovo-vegetarians will eat eggs and dairy products in addition to plant food. If they don't eat eggs, they are *lacto-vegetarians*. If they don't eat dairy products, they are *ovo-vegetarians*.

Fruitarians There are generally two types of fruitarians: those who eat only the things we think of as fruits and those who include nuts under the label of fruits.

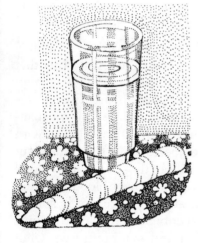

History: Vegetarians tend to have fewer of the major diseases. Those who eat animal fats such as cheese, milk, etc., have a greater risk of heart disease, cancer, etc., than strict vegans and fruitarians. However, vegetarians who eat dairy products and eggs are much more likely to stay young, healthy and sexy than people on the typical American diet. Being vegetarian does not *necessarily* make your diet a healthy one if it is chock-full of candy, alcohol, coffee, cokes, processed foods, etc. Generally, vegetarians are very food-conscious and eat healthy foods. You can be a vegetarian, for example, and follow the macrobiotic or the Pritikin diet faithfully if you want to do so.

Specifically, What Foods Are Good For Me?

Foods that are high in complex carbohydrates should form the basic foundation for your long-life nutritional program. This includes almost all of the members of the plant kingdom! The variety of gourmet dishes that you can experience when you get away from standard steak and potatoes is, as today's youth so eloquently put it, "awesome"!

Five Long-Life Food Groups
From Which Modern-Day Methuselahs
Select 80% Of Their Food

Food Group | **Partial List of Long-Life Foods**

---

1. **VEGETABLES** Most vegetables can be considered long-life foods. They are low in calories, high in fiber, have small but significant amounts of protein and contain vitamins and minerals. Avoid all canned vegetables containing salt, sugar and other additives. Preference should be given to fresh rather than frozen vegetables. The vegetables below are especially nutritious:

Asparagus	Beets
Beet Greens	Broccoli
Brussels Sprouts	Red Cabbage
Cabbage	Chinese Cabbage
Carrots	Cauliflower
Celery	Collards
Cucumbers	Dandelion Greens
Eggplant	Escarole
Endive	Kale
Bib Lettuce	Boston Lettuce
Red Lettuce	Romaine Lettuce
Mushrooms	Mustard Greens
Okra	Onions
Parsley	Parsnips
Peas	Green Peppers
Pumpkin	White Potatoes
Radishes	Rutabagas
Scallions	Spinach
Sweet Potatoes	Tomatoes
Turnips	Turnip Greens

Food Group	Partial List of Long-Life Foods

2. GRAINS

Eat only whole grains. *Whole grains* are those in which the outer shell or husk has been removed but the nutrients and fiber remain virtually untouched. In comparison, "enriched white flour" is basically starch. Twenty-four essential nutrients are removed in the refining process, while only four are added back in to "enrich" it. The less processing grain or flour has undergone, the better it is for you.

Whole-grain cereals are the most nutritious. Avoid like the plague all cereals that contain sugar.

Bread that is made without salt, sugar or other sweeteners, fats or oils, preservatives and additives, whole milk or whole eggs, and is made from 100% stone-ground whole grains is the most nutritious. The idea is to get the maximum nutrition and flavor from the grain without added fat, sugar, salt, and artificial ingredients.

Pasta should be made from whole grains or vegetables. Pasta made from spinach, Jerusalem artichoke and whole wheat is generally available. The grains and grain products listed below are especially nutritious:

Pearled Barley	Corn
Corn Bread	Cream of Rye
Oatmeal	Rye and Flax Cereal
Millet	Whole-Wheat Bread
Rye Bread	Oatmeal Bread
All-Grain Sprouts	Sprouted-Grain
Brown Rice	Breads
Shredded Wheat	

Food Group	Partial List of Long-Life Foods

3. **BEANS & PEAS**

Dried beans and peas are extremely rich sources of protein, minerals and vitamins. Beans and peas vary in their fat content. Pritikin limits people to about 1½ pounds per week (cooked). Macrobiotic diets include beans as a regular staple accounting for about 10% of the food consumed. The beans and peas below are especially nutritious in both dried and sprouted form:

Chickpeas	Chickpea Sprouts
Black-eyed Peas	Black Beans
Brown Beans	Pinto Beans
Kidney Beans	Red Mexican Beans
Navy Beans	Pea Beans
Lentils	Lima Beans
String Beans	Green Peas

4. **FRUITS**

Fruits are an excellent source of vitamins, minerals, fiber and proteins. Some experts say that fruitarians have the healthiest diet. The only difficulty with the diet is consuming enough calories! There are two fruits that are high in fat: olives and avocados. They should be eaten in moderation. You can eat all the fresh fruit you want. Stay away from canned fruit; most of it contains additives and sugar. Sun-dried fruits are fine but higher in calories. Frozen fruits without added sugar are okay. The fruits below are especially good for you and good to eat. It is assumed that all of the juices mentioned are unsweetened.

Apples	Apple Juice
Applesauce	Baked Apples
Apricots	Dried Apricots
Bananas	Baked Bananas
Blackberries	Blueberries
Cantaloupe	Cherries

Food Group	Partial List of Long-Life Foods

Cranberries	Grapefruit Juice
Grapefruit	Grape Juice
Grapes	Guavas
Honeydew Melon	Lemon Juice
Lemons	Lime Juice
Limes	Mango Juice
Mangoes	Muskmelons
Oranges	Orange Juice
Papayas	Papaya Juice
Peaches	Peach Juice
Raisins	Dried Figs
Figs	Prunes
Raspberries	Strawberries
Watermelon	Pineapple

5. **CONDIMENTS**   Avoid all dressings containing sugar, oil, salt, egg yolks and fat. You can use any spice you want as long as it is not premixed with salt. Raw apple-cider vinegar and white wines without additives may be used in dressings. Lemon juice works well too. You will probably have to make your own dressings. Even the ones sold in health-food stores contain sugar (honey), salt (sea salt) and fats (cold-pressed oil).

But What about My Favorite Foods?

Psycholgically, it is difficult for anyone to make a total switch to even the best-pre-pared meals if they are decidedly different from what you've been eating for years. The answer to the problem, both nutri-tionally and psychologically, is to practice common-sense moderation. The chart below spells out exactly how modern-day Methuselahs practice moderation in their eating habits.

Seven Short-Life Food Groups
That Modern-Day Methuselahs Use In Moderation

Food Group	Approach

1. DAIRY PRODUCTS

Some people are allergic to dairy products. Some experts make a very strong case for avoiding cow's milk altogether since it is very different from human mother's milk and has a particularly high fat content. If you are going to use milk products, do so in moderation. Use only low-fat versions and remember that these count as part of your maximum intake of fat.

You can eat in moderation: Skim milk, nonfat milk, nonfat cheeses made from 100% skim milk, buttermilk made with a fat content of 1% or less, and yogurt made from skim milk.

Stay away from: Cream, whole milk, regular buttermilk, full-fat yogurt and cheeses.

2. EGGS

The whites of eggs are okay if you want to get your protein from animal sources, but the yolks of eggs are high in fat.

3. MEAT AND POULTRY

The meat and poultry in this country is contaminated with hormones, antibiotics, preservatives, artificial colorings and flavorings. Not only that, meat is not high on the list of long-life foods. It is too high in saturated fat and doesn't have fiber or carbohydrates. It has few vitamins and minerals. It takes too long to move through our digestive tract, which allows the toxic products of meat digestion to enter our systems. Meat is high in protein. This puts excessive demands on the kidneys and creates increased uric acid in the blood and calcium loss. Research has shown that all these factors are directly or indirectly related to increased risk of bowel cancer, among other things.

You can eat in moderation: Lean beef, turkey and chicken without the skin. Think of meat as a condiment. Don't eat more than 2 or 3 ounces per day. Allow yourself to explore other foods.

Stay away from: Geese, ducks, lamb, mutton, all organ meats, and other fatty meats like bacon, hot dogs, spareribs, sausages, luncheon meats, etc.

4. **FISH**

Fish are not treated with hormones and other additives; however, they absorb toxins from polluted waters. Some fish, especially shellfish, are as high in cholesterol as lamb and beef. Like meat, fish is high in protein. This puts excessive demands on the kidneys, creates increased uric acid in the blood and increases calcium loss. Many large ocean-going fish accumulate excessive amounts of toxins and heavy metals and have been found to have cancer. There is some evidence that cancer can be transmitted from one species to another by ingesting the flesh.

You can eat in moderation: White-fleshed ocean fish such as snapper, sea bass, sole and cod. Clams and lobster are okay once in a while in very small portions. Eat fish as a condiment as the Japanese do.

Stay away from: Large ocean fish like swordfish, tuna and shark, and all shellfish other than clams and lobster and oily fish.

5. **NUTS, SEEDS**

Generally speaking, nuts are a good source of complete protein. Unlike meat, they are not high in cholesterol or saturated fats (except for coconuts). They have several drawbacks, however. Nuts and seeds range from 45 to 90% fat. They are also high in calories. A cup of peanuts is over 800 calories, while a cup of strawberries is only 55 calories. Because of their high oil content, nuts can go rancid quickly.

Eat nuts in moderation. The high-calorie, high-fat content of nuts and seeds puts them in the category of a once-in-a-while treat. Eat nuts from shells to avoid the risk of eating rancid ones.

Stay away from: Salted and roasted nuts and seeds in plastic bags, cans and jars. The only way to make sure they are fresh is to crack them yourself!

6. **DESSERTS**

Desserts are a no-no if they are made from anything resembling refined sugar. This includes sucrose, fructose, maple syrup, corn syrup, etc. You can, however, make desserts from fruits that are nutritious and that will not give you the "sugar rush" that leads to hypoglycemia and other serious complications.

Eat in moderation: Desserts made from cooked fruits and whole grains. An occasional journey into your old habits won't kill you if you have the ability to go back to healthy eating without guilt feelings the next day.

Stay away from all sugars.

7. **BUTTER AND OILS**

Butter, margarine, corn oil, soy oil, peanut oil, safflower oil, etc., are all fats. They are high in calories and low in fiber. A diet high in fats increases your risk of getting cancer, heart disease, diabetes and gout.

Eat in moderation: Very small amounts of oil and butter for stir-frying and sautéing. Count the calories of these fats in your total allotment of fat. Recent research suggests that olive oil may be the best oil to use because it protects you from heart disease. Remember, however, that it is pure fat, and use it sparingly.

Stay away from: All fried foods and foods cooked in oil or butter.

How Do I Find Healthy Food?

Shopping for nutritious, healthy food can be frustrating because things are not always what they appear to be. This is because food manufacturers, processors and distributors spend tons of money studying what people will buy at what price. Just going to a health-food store will not necessarily keep you from purchasing food that is too high in sugar or fat. Last week we bought some "100% whole-wheat fig squares" in one of the health-food stores where we shop. When we got home and read the label, we realized that the contents were not the same as the brand we usually buy at another health-food store. They contained four varieties of refined sugar: honey, barley malt, maple syrup and corn syrup. All this was billed under the heading "no preservatives, no artificial ingredients, 100% whole-wheat and figs"! The chart below will get you started on learning how to read labels so that you can protect yourself from buying food that is not good for you.

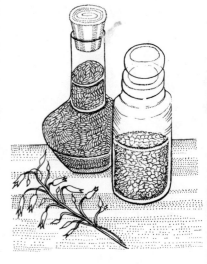

Six Ways Food Processors Trick You With Labels

Their Label	What's The Scoop?
1. Enriched wheat flour	**This is not a whole-grain flour.** It is another name for highly processed, refined white flour.
2. Corn syrup, high-fructose corn syrup, corn sweeteners, maple syrup, fructose, dextrose, sucrose and honey	**Just other names for refined sugar.**
3. Safflower oil, corn oil, coconut oil, peanut oil and olive oil, partially and fully hydrogenated shortening, margarine, butter, lard, beef fat and chicken fat	**Pure fat!** Note that products labeled "no cholesterol" are not necessarily low in fat.
4. "High energy," "lite," "natural," "measurable"	**Advertising labels that are essentially meaningless.** Foods labeled "high energy" are usually high in calories and not in nutrients. Foods labeled "lite" may or may not have fewer calories. They may just be "fluffier" or lighter in color!
5. "No cholesterol," "no preservatives"	**Doesn't tell what is really there!** These labels are used to entice you to buy the product. Read the label. While the product may not contain cholesterol or preservatives, it may very well contain other harmful ingredients, such as high fat, salt, sugar, food colors, etc.
6. "Buttery," "light butter taste," "fortified"	**These labels mean there's no butter!** This type of label is used so you'll buy the product. Similar labels are around for cheese ("cheesy flavor"). The question you should ask of the "fortified" label is "Fortified with what?" The quality and quantity of the vitamins added probably aren't worth the price or even necessary. In many cases "fortifying" bread is an attempt to replace the natural vitamins they took out when they refined and bleached the flour!

Learn to read the labels with a great deal of skepticism, even in health-food stores.

Are There Some Rules I Can Follow In Selecting My Foods?

The best way to get healthy food without additives or preservatives is to grow your own! Unfortunately, for many of us, this is only a dream. The next best thing is to look for foods in your local supermarkets, health-food stores and farm stands that meet the following criteria:

Seven Criteria For Selecting Food To Eat

Criteria	Reasons for Selection
1. **LOW FAT**	People who eat low-fat diets have a lower risk of heart disease and cancer. Select foods that are less than 20% fat. Pritikin's books have extensive lists of foods and their respective fat content. Remember your total fat intake should not exceed 10% of your total calories. Don't fall into the trap of ordering a salad that may have a total of 100 calories in the vegetables and topping it off with an oil-based dressing that has 100 calories per tablespoon. You could end up with 85% of your calories for that meal as fat. Some examples of foods whose ingredients are 20% fat or less:

Skim Milk	Farmer's Cheese
Uncreamed Cottage Cheese	Most Grains
	Most Vegetables
Pasta	Cereals
Fruit	Broiled Ocean
Dried Beans	Perch

2. **HIGH FIBER FOOD**   People who have a shortage of fiber in their diet suffer from increased rates of coronary artery disease, colon cancer, diabetes, diverticular disease and obesity. Fiber helps keep cholesterol from building up in arteries. It speeds cancer-causing materials through the digestive tract. It has no calories and regulates the bowels. Some foods with lots of fiber:

All Dried Beans	Fresh Lima Beans
Fresh Green Peas	Fresh Corn
Figs	Apricots
Strawberries	Raspberries
Blackberries	Dates
Broccoli	Potatoes with skin
Plums with skin	Pears with skin
Apples with skin	Bananas
Carrots	Brussels Sprouts
Spinach	Beet Greens
Collards	Kale
Turnip Greens	Swiss Chard
Raisins	Prunes
Almonds	Peanuts
Walnuts	Brazil Nuts
Whole Wheat	Whole Rye
Whole Oats	Buckwheat
Stone-ground Corn	All breads, rolls, etc., made with whole grains

3. **COMPLEX, UNREFINED CARBOHYDRATES**   Do not confuse complex carbohydrates (starches) with simple carbohydrates (sugars). Sugars are mostly empty calories, while unrefined complex carbohydrates are an almost perfect source of energy. In addition to containing lots of fiber, these foods are extremely nourishing and filling without being fattening. All unprocessed whole grains, fresh vegetables and fruits fit into this category. Take your pick!

4. **NATURALLY FERMENTED**   Fermented foods, such as sauerkraut and yogurt, are partially digested foods which have been broken down naturally by living

organisms. Because they are predigested, they are easily assimilated by the body. They are extremely rich in lactobacillus bacteria, which is good for your digestion. In addition, they contain valuable enzymes and predigested protein.

Cultures known for long life use much fermented food, e.g., yogurt, soured milk, sourdough bread. Watch out for so-called fermented vegetable foods that have been fermented using vinegar instead of the natural fermentation process. Pickles and sauerkraut should contain only the vegetables with some salt. You can also find these foods in salt-free varieties.

5. **FREE OF ADDITIVES, CHEMICALS, PRESERVATIVES**

The long-term effects of eating food containing dyes, food coloring, preservatives, pesticides and other chemicals are not known. In addition, many people are allergic to artificial ingredients. People from long-lived cultures do not eat food with additives or preservatives. Many additives have been shown to cause cancer and tumors in laboratory animals. Dr. James A. O'Shea, who runs the Environmental Medicine Clinic in Lawrence, Massachusetts, has had tremendous success in treating allergies caused by the chemicals in our food, water and air. The field of environmental medicine is growing, and you may want to look for a similar clinic near your home to determine how various forms of pollution are affecting your mental and physical well-being.

6. **ORGANICALLY GROWN, NATURAL**

By natural food we mean food that is grown in fertile soil without chemical fertilizers, pesticides or herbicides. While this is a controversial topic, the logic behind it makes sense. People from long-lived cultures eat food that is grown organically.

If you cannot find this kind of food, ask your physician about taking supplements to protect yourself from the effects of the poisons in your food.

7. **PURE WATER ONLY**   The fact that our natural resources, including soil and water, are becoming increasingly contaminated with industrial waste, runoffs from chemical farming methods, etc., is no longer in dispute. Almost every supermarket in the country now sells bottled spring and mineral water. If you don't have your own supply of fresh spring or well water, find a way to purchase it. Don't rely on the label. Investigate and have it tested. Your own city or town water may be better than some of the bottled water sold by unscrupulous wholesalers. If you have your own water supply, periodically have it tested for purity.

Do I Have To Become A Vegetarian?

No you don't have to become a full-fledged vegetarian. You can stay young, healthy and sexy without becoming a vegetarian if you get 80% of your calories from unrefined carbohydrates and about 10% each from fat and protein.

What Is The Case For Eating Less Meat?

Scientific research comparing vegetarians of all varieties to meat eaters can be summarized as follows:

Disease Area	Findings
1. **CANCER**	a. Worldwide, the incidence of breast, colon and prostate cancer in vegetarians is less than half that in meat eaters.

Disease Area	Findings

b. These types of cancer are practically nonexistent in underdeveloped countries where people live on low-fat, low-protein, high-carbohydrate diets.

2. **HEART DISEASE AND HIGH BLOOD PRESSURE**

a. Vegetarians have significantly lower levels of cholesterol in their blood. When a group of vegetarians were fed eight ounces of meat a day for four weeks, their blood cholesterol rose 19% even though their weight did not increase.

b. Vegetarians have a significantly lower risk of heart disease.

c. Vegetarians have significantly lower blood pressure. A recent study of a group of vegetarians found that only 2% had high blood pressure as compared to 26% of the nonvegetarian control group.

3. **OBESITY, GOUT DIABETES, OSTEOPOROSIS**

a. On the average, vegetarians are thinner and weigh less than meat eaters. A recent study found that only 15% of vegetarians are overweight, while 40% of average, meat-eating Americans are overweight.

b. The incidence of diabetes and gout is significantly lower in vegetarians.

c. In the group of vegetarians who eat no animal fat at all and don't eat eggs or dairy products, adult-onset diabetes and obesity are extremely rare conditions. There is also a considerably lower incidence of osteoporosis in older vegans.

Are There Any Foods I Should Really Pay Attention To?

If you eat a wide variety of fruits, vegetables and grains, the chances of your having health problems due to poor nutrition are slim. This assumes, of course, that you do not exceed the 10% fat, 10 to 12% protein rule of thumb. There are, however, some foods that may provide protection for you against some of the diseases that plague our society today.

Selected Foods That Protect You From Disease

Foods	Did You Know?
1. **APRICOTS, CANTA-LOUPES, CARROTS, PEACHES, SPINACH, TOMATOES**	These foods contain significant amounts of vitamin A, better known as beta-carotene. Beta-carotene protects against cancer of the larynx, lungs, and esophagus. Researchers have found that when people ate two carrots every morning for three weeks, their cholesterol levels went down 11% and their bowels increased the elimination of bile acid and fats by 50%.
2. **BRUSSEL SPROUTS, BROCCOLI, KALE, CABBAGE, COLLARDS, CAULIFLOWER, KOHLRABI**	These are foods from the cabbage family, which research shows can protect against cancer of the stomach, bowels, colon and lungs. In tests with animals, they have been shown to be particularly effective against cancers produced by chemicals.
3. **FISH OIL**	Recent research suggests that fish oils can protect against heart disease and stroke.
4. **OLIVE OIL**	Olive oil, a monounsaturated fat, helps to lower the levels of "bad" cholesterol (low-density lipoprotein) while leaving the "good"

Selected Foods That Protect You From Disease

Foods	Did You Know?
	cholesterol (high-density lipoprotein) alone. Olive oil protects against heart disease and blood clots.
5. **APPLES, PEARS**	Apples and pears are high in fiber and pectin. Research has shown that pectin absorbs cholesterol, thus increasing its elimination from your system. "An apple a day...!"
6. **BANANAS**	Bananas are one of the best desserts you can have. Although they are low in calories, they are one of the most complete foods. Low in salt and 99.8% fat-free, they are excellent for low-sodium and low-fat diets. Bananas contain beta-carotene and vitamin C, both anti-cancer nutrients. They are also high in potassium, which is good for your blood sugar and your heart.
7. **GARLIC, ONIONS**	First cousins, garlic and onions help to lower blood cholesterol and protect against blood clotting and heart disease.
8. **OATS**	Remember when your mother insisted that oatmeal was good for you? She was right. Research has demonstrated that oats help control your cholesterol levels and protect you against heart disease. Oats have more nutrients than wheat or corn.
9. **WHOLE-GRAIN BROWN RICE**	Whole-grain brown rice is an exceptionally nutritious food. It contains high-quality protein and complex carbohydrates. Brown rice protects against cancer and diabetes.

CHAPTER TWELVE WORKSHEET

Long-term Goal(s) _____ Rewards _____

_____

_____

_____

_____

_____

_____

_____

_____

Short-term Goals _____ Rewards _____

_____

_____

_____

_____

_____

_____

_____

_____

_____

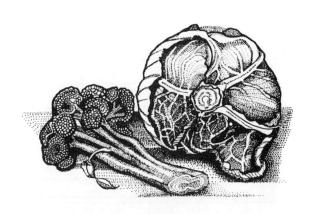

NOTES

The Psychology Of Modifying Your Eating Habits

How Do I Modify My Eating Habits?

We want to make something very clear: This chapter is not about how to lose weight. Weight-loss diets are notoriously unsuccessful. Although some people manage to lose weight on weight-loss diets, 90% gain it all back within a year. This is not good for you either physically or psychologically!

This chapter will teach you how to modify your eating habits permanently so that you will eat and enjoy foods that help you stay young, healthy and sexy! You don't count calories when you are eating for long life and health. If you are getting 80% of your calories from complex carbohydrates, you can eat as much as you want of these foods. Just make sure you watch your fat and protein intake.

You don't count calories when you eat for long life and health.

Although our eating modification program is health motivated, not weight-loss motivated, you will lose weight without counting calories or going hungry – if you stick to the guidelines of 80% complex carbohydrates, 10% fat and 10% protein.

1. **SET A VERY SPECIFIC LONG-TERM MODIFICATION GOAL THAT YOU CAN MEASURE**

   Example:
   At the end of three months from today, I will no longer drink coffee or any other beverage that contains caffeine.

2. **BREAK YOUR LONG-TERM GOAL INTO SHORT-TERM GOALS THAT YOU CAN ACHIEVE RIGHT AWAY**

   Examples:
   Tomorrow morning I will drink only one cup of coffee with breakfast.

   Beginning next Monday, I will drink only one cup of coffee with each meal, with a maximum of three cups per day.

   Beginning two weeks from Monday, I will drink only one cup of coffee per day with one of my meals.

   The problem with eliminating some foods from your diet is that it can leave a real gap in your life. For example, some people use a cup of coffee as a time to relax. Going for a drink after work is an opportunity to socialize with people from the office. Dessert is often viewed as a reward. If you simply eliminate these things without finding a replacement, you'll soon feel deprived. So, try to find acceptable substitutes. Water-processed decaffeinated coffee doesn't contain the chemicals of chemically-processed decaffeinated coffee. Try some of the herb teas. Hot water with lemon is surprisingly tasty. Order a Virgin Mary (a Bloody Mary without the vodka) or bubbly water and lime. Don't give up desserts. Make an effort to find acceptable alternatives, such as baked apples (without sugar) or fresh strawberries or air-popped popcorn.

3. **REWARD YOURSELF IMMEDIATELY WITH SOMETHING YOU LIKE**

Examples:

A new magazine to read.

A chance to read a book you have been wanting to read for a long time.

Calling up some friends and going to the movies on impulse.

4. **MAKE SURE THE REWARD DOES NOT CONFLICT WITH GOOD EATING HABITS**

Example of Conflicting Reward:

A hot-fudge sundae.

Examples of Appropriate Rewards:

A baked apple with cinnamon.

A new murder mystery.

On Rewards:

We cannot overemphasize that **you** must pick the reward and that you must reward yourself **continuously and immediately** in the beginning. The rewards that someone else would choose for you may not be motivating to you, only to them.

5. **CHANGE THE SCENE OF YOUR BAD EATING HABITS**

Example:

Don't allow yourself to snack in front of the TV or in the bedroom. Allow yourself to eat only in the kitchen.

6. **CHALLENGE YOURSELF TO EAT HEALTHY FOODS**

Examples:

Decide to look younger and have more energy next year than you do now.

Decide to master the basic facts of long-life nutrition so that you can help others in your family.

7. **LEARN TO EAT HEALTHY FOODS FROM SOMEONE WHO HAS ALREADY MODIFIED HIS OR HER EATING HABITS**

Examples:

Join a health club and look for new friends who have successfully rejuvenated themselves.

Read stories of people who have overcome serious health problems and have subsequently become vibrant, healthy and active people through good nutrition and exercise.

7. **GET YOUR LOVED ONES INVOLVED IN YOUR PROGRAM TO MODIFY YOUR EATING HABITS**

Examples:

Get your spouse to work with you to develop a schedule for gradually eliminating sugar from the family diet.

Ask your friend to remind you (gently and quietly) every time you eat candy.

8. **EVALUATE AND REEVALUATE YOUR PROGRESS**

Example:

Every time you slip back into an old habit (i.e., eating a candy bar), talk to yourself (and others) about it. Try to figure out a way to avoid the stimulus that brought on that response. If it was a stress-related response, then have an acceptable snack (like an apple) ready the next time it happens.

9. **SEE YOURSELF AS YOUNG, HEALTHY AND SEXY, GAINING YOUR VITALITY FROM GOOD NUTRITION**

Examples:

Create an image of yourself growing younger as each day passes. See yourself eating healthy food that causes this to happen. Keep this vision before you when you daydream or meditate (see Chapter 7 on visualization).

Every morning when you wake up, take a moment to look in the mirror. Say to yourself, "Every day in every way I'm getting younger, more in control of myself, more powerful..."

10. **POST A LIST OF YOUR GOALS**

Example:

Hang a list of your goals over your desk and bathroom mirror.

Making The Move To Long-Life Nutrition

As we mentioned earlier, modifying your eating habits means modifying some of your feelings about food. When we began to switch to a more healthy nutritional program, we found ourselves constantly sliding back into our old "happiness is eating certain foods" habits. (e.g., ice cream is a reward for good work).

One of the ways we prevented too many backsliding incidents was to get the "bad" food out of our kitchen. This really took some doing since we had invested a considerable amount of our hard-earned money in packaged, canned and processed food that we were rapidly discovering were not healthy for us. We decided that in the long run it was probably much less costly to throw food out now than to pay medical bills in the future. We found that once we accepted the fact that we had to modify the kind of food we purchased, it became a challenge. Since the day we literally emptied out our kitchen, our motto has been, "Don't change what you eat; change the quality of what you eat." That's our first tip. If you are going to make the switch to more nutritious food, start with the food-quality problem. Then move on to more extensive modifications. A good example of the quality-substitution approach is to buy a brand name of ketchup called "Un-ketchup," which contains no salt and no sugar, only tomatoes, spices and apple juice. The manufacturers are prohibited from calling it ketchup because the law requires sugar in ketchup!

Don't change what you eat, change the quality and relative proportions of what you eat.

1. **TAKE IT SLOW** Take it slow and easy. Modifying your eating habits should be done bit by bit.

2. **IT'S OKAY TO BACKSLIDE** When you fall back into an old habit, don't use it as an excuse to go back to your old ways permanently. You will have plenty of backsliding days. They will get less frequent over time, but the habit won't go away instantly. Don't feel guilty. Just begin again the next day.

3. **SET AN EXAMPLE** Don't bore other people with your new-found "superior information." Set an example. Let them observe how much more energy you have, how much more productive you are, how much weight you have lost, how young you look, etc. When they ask you, then tell them about it, a little at a time.

4. **TAPER OFF FROM FAT AND PROTEIN GRADUALLY** Get rid of high-fat, high-protein meals. If you want to keep meat in your diet, your long-term goal should be to use it as a condiment.

5. **THROW AWAY THE SALT SHAKER** Get rid of it now! You don't need it. Stay away from fast foods and pickles. There are some pretty good salt-free pickles around. Substitute foods that are fermented without salt.

6. **BREAK THE SUGAR ADDICTION** Make a concerted effort to taper off your use of refined sugar. First, gradually eliminate it from your cooking and substitute other sweeteners like honey or maple syrup. The ideal goal is to get rid of all highly refined sweeteners, one at a time, starting with white sugar. We now use cooked apples or mashed ripe bananas to sweeten our oatmeal. Delicious!

7.	**WHOLE GRAINS ONLY**	Substitute whole-wheat flour and whole grain breads for white flour. This is a fairly easy substitution because 100% stone-ground whole wheat has much more flavor than bleached and refined white flour.
8.	**ELIMINATE CAFFEINE**	This means no cokes or similar beverages, coffee, tea or chocolate. Carob makes an excellent and healthy substitute for chocolate. There are dozens of herb teas. Perrier or Poland Spring water with a fresh lime or lemon twist are excellent substitutes for alcoholic and caffeine beverages. There are a number of grain coffee substitutes. There is also Swiss water-processed decaffeinated coffee. It supposedly doesn't contain the bad chemcials of other decafs. We risk it once a day but are carefully watching the research on this one!
9.	**LEARN TO COOK AND EAT DIFFERENTLY**	Learn to prepare your food in healthy ways. Learn to steam lightly rather than boil. Learn to eat a lot of raw food, salads without oil-based dressings, fruit, etc. Snack on fruit, carrots and celery. Eat your food in the right order. High protein foods like dairy, fish and tofu should be eaten first. Then eat the faster moving foods such as grains, steamed greens, raw vegetables and fruits so that they help to push the slower-moving proteins through your system more quickly. This means that when you go out to eat, you eat your salad last.
10.	**EXERCISE**	Research on the relationship between exercise and body weight overwhelmingly supports the need for exercise. You burn up calories when you exercise and **you actually eat less** when you exercise than when you don't!

CHAPTER THIRTEEN WORKSHEET

Long-term Goal(s) _____ Rewards _____

_____

_____

_____

_____

_____

_____

_____

Short-term Goals _____ Rewards _____

_____

_____

_____

_____

_____

_____

_____

_____

_____

_____

_____

_____

Reminder Notes: _____

_____

_____

_____

_____

_____

_____

CHAPTER FOURTEEN

The Latest Research On Vitamins

Why Should I Take Supplements?*

To take or not to take supplements is a controversial issue. In spite of many years of scientific and clinical investigation, we still have a long way to go before we can answer this question with a great deal of certainty. Theoretically, no one who is eating a balanced diet containing a wide variety of foods should require vitamin or mineral supplements. Yet millions of jars of vitamins and minerals are sold every day.

We believe, as many others do, that there are a number of factors in our modern world that prevent us from getting the kind of nutrition that we need to stay young, healthy and sexy from the food that we purchase. Some of the arguments are presented in the chart on the following page.

*WARNING: Do not take food supplements without the approval of your physician or nutritionist.

263

What's Wrong With Our Environment
From A Nutritional Perspective?

Problem	Cause	Result
Depleted soil	Poor agricultural methods Poor land management	Food deficient in important nutrients
Refined foods	Processing in order to make food last longer	Food depleted of optimal nutrients
Food not fresh	Food shipped coast to coast and sold long after the optimal freshness date	Nutritional content depleted
Pollution	Payoff for industrialization: polluted water, soil, air	Toxins in the environment as well as in the food
Food additives, chemicals in food	Preservatives, waxes, fertilizers, fungicides, pesticides, coloring agents and artificial flavorings	Body can't process food properly
Stress	Sources range from fast pace of modern world to work problems to environmental noise to CRT radiation	Body robbed of essential nutrients

Fortunately, scientists have been accumulating more and more evidence that taking vitamin and mineral supplements can protect you from the effects of our increasingly stressful environment. We think of a vitamin and mineral supplementation program as an insurance policy. Healthy people probably can take a high-quality multivitamin on their own without supervision. Anything beyond that requires medical/nutritional supervision by a professional.

This chapter provides you with information about those supplements that are used to

264

protect you from psychological and physical stress. Since we are not nutritionists, this chapter only gives you a brief overview of a very complex field. We strongly urge you to seek the help of a qualified nutritionist to help you pin-point your own individual supplementation needs.

ANTISTRESS VITAMINS

Vitamins that are soluble in water are rapidly used up by the body when it is under stress. Ironically, these same vitamins are the ones you need the most when the going gets tough!

The B Vitamins

So far scientists have identified eleven B vitamins. If you decide to supplement your diet with vitamins, B vitamins should be taken together in a balanced formula. Don't fool around with your own combination of B vitamins. Eat a wide variety of natural foods that are rich in these vitamins.

Vitamin B1: Thiamine

Thiamine is known as the anti-aging vitamin. It is essential for protein metabolism and transforming glucose into energy.

Positive Checklist for Vitamin B1
(Thiamine)
Solubility: Water   Min. Daily Req.: 1 to 1.5 mg.

---

* Anti-aging vitamin

* Protects heart muscle

* Promotes growth

* Aids digestion and peristalsis

* Helps relieve constipation

* Protects you against the effects of lead-poisoning

* Prevents fluid retention

* Prevents fatigue

* Increases stamina

* Aids muscle tone of stomach, intestines

Vitamin B1, thiamine, can be found in a wide variety of plant and animal sources. As part of the effort to eliminate fat and reduce cholesterol, the preference would be to rely on vegetarian sources of B1.

**Natural Food Sources of Vitamin B1
(Thiamine)**

Vegetarian	Animal
Asparagus	*Lacto*
Brewer's yeast	Cheese
Cabbage	Yogurt
Carrots	Milk
Celery	
Coconuts	
Grapefruit	
Lemons	*Meat*
Nuts	Organs
Parsley	Pork
Pineapple	

Vegetarian	Animal
Radishes	
Rice polishings	
Seeds	
Wheat germ	
Whole grain	
Whole-grain cereals	
Watercress	

Vitamin B1 helps your body get rid of the acids that are formed when your system converts glucose into energy. When there is a shortage of vitamin B1, the acid by-products of the sugar breakdown can result in an accumulation of toxic acids in the brain, acid irritation of the heart muscle and nerve cell damage. Severe deficiency can cause beriberi, neuritis, and edema.

Facts About Vitamin B1

Symptoms of Deficiency	Symptoms of Overdose	Things That Use The Vitamin Up Too Fast
Loss of appetite	Same as the	Alcohol
Slow heart beat	symptoms of B	Tobacco
Chronic constipation	complex deficiency.	Coffee
Irritability	See warning note	Surgery
Diabetes	below.	Sugar
Depression		Processed foods
Nervous exhaustion		Raw clams
Poor lactation		Refined foods
Intestinal disorders		
Gastric disorders		
Forgetfulness		
Fatigue		
Shortness of breath		
Pain sensitivity		

Since vitamin B1 is a water-soluble vitamin, the excess beyond what your body needs is excreted in the urine and does not normally build up. At this time, scientists have not identified a toxic dose for vitamin B1.

Warning: Any B vitamin taken out of proportion to all other B vitamins or taken alone can cause depletion and symptoms of deficiency in all the other B vitamins, since they are excreted along with the excess B1. In other words, if you took only B1, without the other B vitamins, you could get the symptoms of deficiency of all of those B vitamins that you are not taking. Therefore, always take all the B vitamins together in a balanced formula.

Vitamin B2: Riboflavin

Riboflavin could be called the anticataract vitamin. It is essential for growth, healthy eyes and general good health.

Positive Checklist for Vitamin B2 (Riboflavin)

Solubility: Water   **Min. Daily Req.: 1.3 to 1.7 mg.**

---

* Promotes healthy eyes, skin

* Promotes healthy nails and hair

* Helps maintain general health

* Protects against some cataracts

* Essential for growth

* Helps thyroid function effectively

Vitamin B2, riboflavin, can be found in a wide variety of plant and animal sources. As part of the effort to eliminate fat and reduce cholesterol, the preference would be to rely on vegetarian sources of vitamin B2.

Natural Food Sources of Vitamin B2 (Riboflavin)

Vegetarian	Animal
Apples	*Lacto*
Apricots	Cheese
Blackstrap molasses	Yogurt
Brewer's yeast	Milk
Cabbage	
Carrots	
Coconuts	
Collards	
Dandelion greens	
Grapefruit	
Prunes	*Meat*
Spinach	Organs
Turnip greens	Pork
Whole-grain cereals	
Watercress	

Vitamin B2 is essential for oxidation and energy release, and aids in protein metabolism and the assimilation of iron. Early signs of deficiency are sores around the mouth, light sensitivity and lack of stamina.

Facts About Vitamin B2

Symptoms of Deficiency	Symptoms of Overdose	Things That Use The Vitamin Up Too Fast
Light sensitivity	Same as the symptoms	Alcohol
Lack of stamina	B-complex deficency.	Tobacco
Digestive disturbances	See warning note on page 268.	

Symptoms of Deficiency	Things That Use The Vitamin Up Too Fast
Cataracts	Coffee
Hair loss	Sugar
Depression	Processed foods
Sore and red tongue	Refined foods
Bloodshot eyes	

Just like vitamin B1, vitamin B2 is a water-soluble vitamin. Therefore, the excess beyond what your body needs is excreted in the urine and does not normally build up. At this time, scientists have not identified a toxic dose for vitamin B2. Remember our warning about the B vitamins. Always take B vitamins together in a balanced formula.

Vitamin B3: Niacin

Niacin is often called the antipellagra vitamin. It is essential for healthy functioning of the nervous system and for proper circulation. It is believed to help prevent migraine headaches and helps maintain healthy skin.

Positive Checklist for Vitamin B3 (Niacin)

Solubility: Water   Min. Daily Req.: 10 to 13 mg.

* Promotes healthy skin

* Promotes proper circulation

* Helps maintain gastrointestinal-tract functions

* May help prevent migraine headaches

* Essential for proper protein and fat metabolism

* Essential for proper carbohydrate metabolism

* Helps reduce cholesterol levels

Vitamin B3, niacin, can be found in a wide variety of plant and animal sources. As part of the effort to eliminate fat and reduce cholesterol, the preference would be to rely on vegetarian sources of B3.

Natural Food Sources of Vitamin B3 (Niacin)

Vegetarian	Animal
Brewer's yeast	*Lacto/Ovo*
Brown rice	Milk Products
Green vegetables	Eggs
Nuts	
Peanuts	
Rice bran	
Rhubarb	*Meat*
Soybeans	Fish
Sunflower seeds	Liver
Torula yeast	Poultry
Wheat germ	
Whole-wheat products	

Vitamin B3, niacin, also goes by other names: niacinamide, nicotinic acid and nicotinic acidomide. The amount of niacin required varies from one person to another.

Facts About Vitamin B3

Symptoms of Deficiency	Symptoms of Overdose	Things That Use The Vitamin Up Too Fast
Unpleasant mouth odor	Red, prickly skin,	Alcohol
Psychological imbalance	liver damage,	Corn
Canker sores	stomach ulcers,	Coffee
Appetite loss	jaundice. See warn-	Sugar
Depression, fatigue	ing note on page	Processed foods
Headaches	268.	Refined foods
Indigestion		Antibiotics
Insomnia		
Nausea		
Skin eruptions		
Muscular weakness		

Just like vitamin B1, vitamin B3 is a water-soluble vitamin. Unlike the other B vitamins, massive doses can cause severe liver damage, peptic ulcers and diabetes. It is not a totally harmless water-soluble vitamin! Also, the individual daily requirement for niacin is considerably higher than that of the other B vitamins. Remember our general warning about the B vitamins. Always take B vitamins together in a balanced formula.

Vitamin B6: Pyridoxine

Pyridoxine could be called the tranquilizer vitamin. It is essential in activating many of the enzymes and enzyme systems and in the production of antibodies to protect you from bacterial diseases. It is also essential to DNA and RNA synthesis. There is some evidence that it may help to prevent bladder cancer.

Positive Checklist for Vitamin B6 (Pyridoxine)

Solubility: Water   Min. Daily Req.: 2.0 to 2.5 mg.

* Helps control weight

* Helps with digestion

* Prevents acne and other skin disorders

* Protects against tooth decay

* Protects against diabetes

* Protects against heart disease

* Protects against bladder cancer

* Helps fight bacterial disease

* Helps maintain sodium-potassium balance

Vitamin B6, pyridoxine, can be found in a wide variety of plant and animal sources. As part of the effort to eliminate fat and reduce cholesterol, the preference would be to rely on vegetarian sources of B6.

Natural Food Sources of Vitamin B6 (Pyridoxine)

Vegetarian	Animal
Avocados	*Lacto/Ovo*
Bananas	Milk
Blackstrap molasses	Egg yolks
Brewer's yeast	
Cabbage	
Cantalope	
Carrots	
Green leafy	*Meat*
vegetables	Desiccated liver
Green peppers	Fish
Peanuts	Organs
Pecans	
Prunes	
Raisins	
Soybeans	
Walnuts	
Wheat bran	
Wheat germ	
Whole grains	

Vitamin B6, pyridoxine, is very effective in treating insomnia because it acts like a tranquilizer. It also helps your body assimilate food. It has been used in the treatment of Parkinson's disease, arthritic and rheumatic conditions, mental retardation, sexual disorders, pancreatitis and hypoglycemia.

Facts About Vitamin B6

Symptoms of Deficiency	Symptoms of Overdose	Things That Use The Vitamin Up Too Fast
Acne, skin disorders	Doses of 150 mg.	Alcohol
Anemia	can cause sleepiness.	Tobacco
Arthritis	Daily doses over 200	Coffee
Irritability	mg. have caused a	Birth-control pills
Hair loss	dependency state after	Radiation exposure
Depression	withdrawal. See	
Learning disabilities	remarks below and	
Weakness	warning note on	
Sore mouth and lips	page 268.	
Bad breath		
Tooth decay		
Migraine headaches		
Premature senility		

Just like vitamin B1, vitamin B6 is a water-soluble vitamin. Therefore, the excess beyond what your body needs is excreted in the urine and does not normally build up. At this time, scientists have not identified the toxic dose for vitamin B6. Remember our warning about the B vitamins. Always take B vitamins together in a balanced formula.

Pantothenic Acid

Pantothenic acid could be called the anti-stress B vitamin. It is essential for the proper utilization of sugar and fat for energy. As stress increases, the body demands increasing amounts of pantothenic acid.

Positive Checklist for Vitamin B5
(Pantothenic Acid)

Solubility: Water   Min. Daily Req.: Not established.
Estimates: 4 to 50 mg.

* Protects against the effects of mental stress

* Protects against the effects of physical stress

* Prevents wrinkles

* Prevents premature aging

* Increases vitality

* Protects against toxins

* Protects against infections

Vitamin B5, pantothenic acid, can be found in a wide variety of plant and animal sources. As part of the effort to eliminate fat and reduce cholesterol, the preference would be to rely on vegetarian sources of B5.

Natural Food Sources of
Pantothenic Acid

Vegetarian	Animal
Beans	*Ovo*
Blackstrap molasses	Egg Yolk
Brewer's yeast	
Cauliflower	
Green vegetables	
Mushrooms	*Meat*
Peas	Liver
Peanuts	Kidneys
Wheat bran	Salmon
Wheat germ	
Whole grains	

Pantothenic acid stimulates the adrenal glands and is essential in maintaining an appropriate level of blood-sugar. It increases your energy and vitality and helps your body ward off infections. It is also an important factor in ensuring a speedy recovery from illness.

Facts About Pantothenic Acid

Symptoms of Deficiency	Symptoms of Overdose	Things That Use The Vitamin Up Too Fast
Low stress resistance	Same as symptoms of	Alcohol
Gray hair	B-complex deficiency.	Tobacco
Stomach distress	See note below and	Coffee
Allergies, asthma	warning on	Sugar
Hair loss	page 268.	Stress
Depression		
Sore and burning feet		
Low blood sugar		
Muscle cramps		
Low blood pressure		
Irritability		
Duodenal ulcer		
Diarrhea		

Scientists have not found any cases of pantothenic acid deficiency. Moreover, they have found it difficult to experimentally induce deficiencies. Just like vitamin B1, pantothenic acid is a water-soluble vitamin. Therefore, the excess beyond what your body needs is excreted in the urine and does not normally build up. At this time, scientists have not identified the toxic dose for vitamin B5. Remember our warning about the B vitamins. Always take B vitamins together in a balanced formula. Pantothenic acid has been used to treat allergies, arthritis, low blood sugar, stress, baldness, infections and tooth decay.

Vitamin H: Biotin

Biotin helps with the metabolism of fats
and protein and is necessary for the utilization of pantothenic acid.

Positive Checklist for Vitamin H
(Biotin)

Solubility: Water   Min. Daily Req.: 150 to 300 mcg.

---

* Promotes healthy hair

* Prevents hair loss

* Helps body use vitamin B-complex

* Can help protect against baldness

* Essential for cell growth

Biotin can be obtained from both plant
and animal sources. As part of the effort
to eliminate fat and reduce cholesterol,
the preference would be to rely on vegetarian sources of biotin.

Natural Food Sources of Vitamin H
(Biotin)

Vegetarian	Animal
Beans	*Lacto/Ovo*
Brewer's yeast	Milk
Mushrooms	Egg yolks
Peanuts	Yogurt
Soybeans	
Unpolished rice	*Meat*
Whole grains	Liver
	Kidneys

Your body can produce biotin in the intestines if there is a sufficient amount of microflora available. Deficiencies of biotin have been produced in laboratory animals. In humans, deficiencies have been produced by the consumption of raw egg whites in **large amounts** (about 20 per day).

Facts About Vitamin H (Biotin)

Symptoms of Deficiency	Symptoms of Overdose	Things That Use The Vitamin Up Too Fast
Dry skin	Actual toxic dose	Alcohol
Depression	unknown. Biotin	Coffee
Fatigue	overdose would have	Raw egg whites
Poor appetite	the same symptoms	Sugar
Lack of stamina	as vitamin B-complex	Antibiotics
Eczema	deficiency. See warn-	Refined food
Hair loss	ing note below and on	Processed food
Dandruff	page 268.	
Seborrhea		
Lung infections		
Heart abnormalities		
Drowsiness		
Hallucinations		
Anemia		

Just like vitamin B1, vitamin H is a water-soluble vitamin. Therefore, the excess beyond what your body needs is excreted in the urine and does not normally build up. At this time, scientists have not identified the toxic dose for biotin. Remember our warning about the B vitamins. Always take B vitamins together in a balanced formula.

Vitamin Bx: PABA
(Para aminobenzoic acid)

PABA could be called the antisunburn vitamin because of its ability to protect you from sunburn and even skin cancer.

PABA is often left out of multiple vitamin compounds because it makes sulfa drugs ineffective.

Positive Checklist for Vitamin Bx
(PABA: Para aminobenzoic acid)

Solubility: Water   **Min. Daily Req.: Not Stated**

---

* Prevents graying of hair

* Promotes healthy skin

* As a salve, helps prevent sunburn

* Promotes growth

* Helps with blood cell formation

PABA can be obtained from both plant and animal sources. As part of the effort to eliminate fat and reduce cholesterol, the preference would be to rely on vegetarian sources of PABA.

Natural Food Sources of Vitamin Bx
(PABA: Para aminobenzoic acid)

Vegetarian	Animal
Brewer's yeast	*Lacto/Ovo*
Molasses	Milk
Wheat germ	Egg yolks
Whole grains	Yogurt
	Meat
	Liver
	Kidneys

Your body can produce PABA in the intestines if there is a sufficient amount of friendly bacteria. Not much is known

about PABA, but it has been used successfully in the treatment of gray hair and is
commonly used as a sunscreen in suntan
lotions and creams.

Facts About Vitamin Bx
(PABA)

Symptoms of Deficiency	Symptoms of Overdose	Things That Use The Vitamin Up Too Fast
Eczema	Toxic dose is 10 to 100	Alcohol
Depression	mg. Dosages over 30	Coffee
Fatigue (extreme)	mg. require a prescrip-	Sulfa drugs
Gray hair	tion. See warning note	Sugar
Anemia	on page 268. Can	
Infertility	cause heart, liver, and	
Reproductive disorders	kidney damage.	
Headaches		
Irritability		
Constipation		
Digestion problems		

Remember our warning about the B vitamins. Always take B vitamins together in
a balanced formula. PABA is not simply a
harmless water-soluble vitamin. Some researchers have reported that high doses
have been toxic to the heart, kidney and
liver.

Vitamin B12: Cobalamin

Cobalamin is known as the red vitamin.
It is essential to the regeneration and production of the red blood cells. Cobalamin
or cyanocobalamin is also important for
proper nerve functioning, helping to
maintain the nerve sheath so that it can
transmit messages.

Positive Checklist for Vitamin B12
(Cobalamin)

Solubility: Water   **Min. Daily Req.: 1 to 5 mcg.**

* Promotes healthy appetite

* Prevents anemia

* Helps nerves function properly

* Promotes growth in children

* Essential for blood-cell growth and longevity

Some experts believe that you cannot get sufficient amounts of B12 from strictly vegetarian sources. This is a controversial issue. Both animal and vegetarian sources are listed in the chart below. Consult your physician.

Natural Food Sources of Vitamin B12
(Cobalamin)

Vegetarian	Animal
Brewer's yeast (fortified)	*Lacto/Ovo* Milk
Comfrey leaves	Eggs
Concord grapes	Yogurt
Cereal (fortified)	Aged cheese
Kelp	Cottage cheese
Peanuts	*Meat*
Raw wheat germ	Chicken
Soy milk (fortified)	Kidneys
Tempeh	Liver
	Trout
	Tuna

Your body can produce vitamin B12 in the intestines if there is a sufficient amount of microflora available. Some nutritionists question whether enough B12 can be provided this way. They claim that strict vegetarians who use no animal products will begin to exhibit deficiency symptoms after five or six years when the B12 stored in the liver is used up. Recent research has not supported this hypothesis.

Facts About Vitamin B12 (Cobalamin)		
Symptoms of Deficiency	**Symptoms of Overdose**	**Things That Use The Vitamin Up Too Fast**
Impaired reflexes	Actual toxic dose unknown. B12 overdose would have the same symptoms as the vitamin B-complex deficiency. See warning note below and on page 268.	Alcohol
Depression		Coffee
Fatigue		Calcium deficiency
Pernicious anemia		B6 deficiency
Weakness in legs/arms		Tobacco
Walking difficulties		Liver disease
Speaking difficulties		Processed food
Memory loss		Laxatives
Nervousness		
Poor concentration		
Sore mouth		
Poor appetite in children		

Just like vitamin B1, vitamin B12 is a water-soluble vitamin. Therefore, the excess beyond what your body needs is excreted in the urine and does not normally build up. At this time, scientists have not identified the toxic dose for colbalamin. Remember our warning about the B vitamins. Always take B vitamins together in a balanced formula.

Vitamin B9: Folic Acid

Folic acid could be called the healing vitamin. It is essential to the healing process, helping to build antibodies which prevent and heal infections. Folic acid works with B12 to help form red blood cells. Also, it works with B12 and vitamin C to help your body break down and use proteins.

Positive Checklist for Vitamin B9
(Folic Acid)

Solubility: Water   **Min. Daily Req.: 400 mcg.**

* Promotes healing process

* Prevents premature gray hair

* Helps form red blood cells

* Essential for reproduction of cells

Folic acid can be found in a variety of foods. As part of the effort to eliminate and reduce cholesterol, the preference would be to rely on vegetarian sources of B9.

Natural Food Sources of Vitamin B9
(Folic Acid)

Vegetarian	Animal
Asparagus	*Lacto/Ovo*
Broccoli	Milk
Dates	Egg
Grapefruit	Yogurt
Green leafy veggies	
Lettuce	*Meat*
Lima beans	Liver
Mushrooms	Oysters
Nuts	Salmon
Oranges	Tuna
Peanuts	
White potatoes	
Spinach	
Whole grains	

Folic acid makes it possible for your body to utilize amino acids and sugar. The division of all of your body cells is partially dependent on its presence. Deficiency can result in serious skin disorders, impaired circulation and loss of hair.

Facts About Vitamin B9 (Folic Acid)		
Symptoms of Deficiency	Symptoms of Overdose	Things That Use The Vitamin Up Too Fast
Hair loss	Actual toxic	Alcohol
Serious skin disorders	dose unknown.	Coffee
Impaired circulation	A B9 overdose	Tobacco
Mental depression	would have the	Sugar
Anemia	same symptoms	Stress
Fatigue	as a vitamin B-	Refined food
Graying hair	complex deficiency.	Processed food
Digestion problems	See warning note	Heat (cooking)
Insomnia	below and on	Sulfa drugs
Tongue inflammation	page 268.	Fever
Memory problems		Birth-control pills
Reproduction problems		
Walking problems		
Speaking problems		

Just like vitamin B1, folic acid is a water-soluble vitamin. Therefore, the excess beyond what your body needs is excreted in the urine and does not normally build up. At this time, scientists have not identified the toxic dose for folic acid. Remember our warning about the B vitamins. Always take B vitamins together in a balanced formula.

Choline

Choline works with inositol (discussed next) as part of lecithin, a substance found naturally in your body. Lecithin helps your body utilize the fat-soluble vitamins, A, D, E and K. Some authorities do not

recognize choline and inositol as vitamins, claiming there is not enough research data to give them the final label.
Others add them to the list that comprises
the B complex.

Positive Checklist for Choline

Solubility: Water   Min. Daily Req.: None Reported

---

* Helps digest blood fats

* Prevents fatty deposits in liver

* Helps body use vitamins A, D, E, K

* Minimizes cholesterol buildup in arteries

* Prevents gallstones

* Reduces high blood pressure

Choline can be obtained from a number
of natural sources. As part of the effort
to eliminate fat and reduce cholesterol,
the preference would be to rely on vegetarian sources of choline.

Natural Food Sources of Choline

Vegetarian	Animal
Brewer's Yeast	*Lacto/Ovo*
Beans	Egg yolks
Green leafy veggies	
Peanuts	*Meat*
Soybeans	Fish
Lecithin	Liver
Wheat germ	Kidneys

If you have a normal, healthy diet, your body can manufacture its own choline. Scientists are not certain what the minimum daily requirements are, but estimates are around 1000 mg. A long-term deficiency can lead to high blood pressure, hardening of the arteries and a buildup of fatty deposits in your liver.

Facts About Choline

Symptoms of Deficiency	Symptoms of Overdose	Things That Use The Vitamin Up Too Fast
Fat intolerance	Actual toxic dose	Alcohol
High blood pressure	unknown. See note	Coffee
Cirrhosis of the liver	below and warning	Sugar
Bleeding stomach ulcers	note on page 268.	
Heart trouble		

Just like vitamin B1, choline is a water-soluble vitamin. Therefore, the excess beyond what your body needs is excreted in the urine and does not normally build up. At this time, scientists have not identified the toxic dose for choline. Remember our warning about the B vitamins. Always take B vitamins together in a balanced formula.

Inositol

Inositol works with choline (discussed above) as part of lecithin, a substance found naturally in your body. Lecithin helps your body utilize the fat-soluble vitamins, A, D, E and K. Some authorities do not recognize inositol and choline as vitamins, claiming there is not enough research data to give them the final label. Others add them to the list that comprises the B complex.

Positive Checklist for Inositol

Solubility: Water   Min. Daily Req.: None Reported

* Essential for hair growth

* Prevents thinning hair and baldness

* Helps reduce blood cholesterol

* Helps maintain a healthy heart muscle

* Helps digest vitamins A, D, E, K

Inositol can be obtained from a number of natural sources. Inositol is one of the most prevalent vitamins in the body but is concentrated in the eyes and the heart. Both animal and vegetable sources are listed in the chart below. As part of the program to eliminate fat and reduce cholesterol, the preference would be to rely on vegetarian sources wherever possible.

Natural Food Sources of Inositol

Vegetarian	Animal
Blackstrap molasses	
Brewer's yeast	*Lacto/Ovo*
Corn	Milk
Grapefruit	Yogurt
Lecithin	
Nuts	*Meat*
Oatmeal	Liver
Oranges	Kidneys
Peanuts	
Wheat germ	
Whole grains	
Vegetables	

According to many researchers, your body is able to synthesize adequate amounts of inositol for your use. Moreover, inositol occurs naturally in large amounts in many common foods. Many experts no longer include it as a vitamin. Scientists are not certain what the minimum daily requirements are, but estimates are generally the same as those for choline. Deficiency can lead to high blood cholesterol, eye problems and constipation.

Facts About Inositol?

Symptoms of Deficiency	Symptoms of Overdose	Things That Use The Vitamin Up Too Fast
High cholesterol Constipation Eczema Eye problems Hair loss	Actual toxic dose unknown. See note below and warning note on page 268.	Alcohol Coffee

---

Just like choline, inositol is a water-soluble vitamin. Therefore, the excess beyond what your body needs is excreted in the urine and does not normally build up. At this time, scientists have not identified the toxic dose for inositol. Remember our warning about the B vitamins. Always take B vitamins together in a balanced formula.

Vitamin C

Like folic acid, Vitamin C could be called the healing vitamin. It promotes healing in all cases of illness, regardless of condition or type. It protects from stress and is a general detoxicant. It is extremely important to the functioning of your body's immune system.

Positive Checklist for Vitamin C
(Ascorbic Acid)

Solubility: Water   Min. Daily Req.: 30 to 70 mg.

* Promotes healing

* Promotes digestion

* Helps body defend against toxins

* Helps you fight emotional stress

* Prevents common colds

* Promotes healthy teeth and gums

* Promotes healthy bones

Ascorbic acid can be obtained from most vegetables and fruits. The sources listed on the chart below represent particularly excellent sources.

Natural Food Sources of Vitamin C
(Ascorbic Acid)

Fruits	Vegetables
Apples	Broccoli
Citrus fruits	Cabbage
Cantalope	Green pepper
Grapefruit	Potatoes
Guavas	Turnip greens
Papaya	
Rose hips	
Strawberries	
Tomatoes	

Your body cannot synthesize vitamin C, so you must obtain it from the food you eat and/or supplements. The most basic function of vitamin C identified so far is its role in forming collagen, a body protein that makes up the tissue in your bones, teeth, skin and muscles. Scurvy, one of the oldest deficiencies known to science, is due to a vitamin-C deficiency.

Facts About Vitamin C
(Ascorbic Acid)

Symptoms of Deficiency	Symptoms of Overdose	Things That Use The Vitamin Up Too Fast
Anemia	Burning on	Antibiotics
Bleeding gums	urination	Aspirin
Breath shortness	Loose bowels	Cortisone
Bruises	Skin rashes	Tobacco
Low resistance to	Kidney stones	Stress
infection	Toxic dose is	
Muscle cramps	5,000 to 15,000 mg.	
Nose bleeds		
Poor digestion		
Scurvy		
Swollen joints		
Tooth decay		

Just like vitamin B1, vitamin C is a water-soluble vitamin. Generally, vitamin C has been thought to be non-toxic and has been used in fairly large doses for the prevention of colds and to aid in healing infections. It is believed that the excess beyond what your body needs is excreted. More recently there has been some evidence that it may cause kidney stones when taken in large dosages. We urge you to consult with your physician or nutritionist before taking large doses over an extended period of time.

CHAPTER FOURTEEN WORKSHEET

Long-term Goal(s)＿＿＿＿＿＿＿＿ Rewards ＿＿＿＿＿＿＿＿

Determine whether or not supplements are needed.

＿＿＿＿＿＿＿＿＿＿＿＿＿＿＿＿＿＿＿＿＿＿＿＿

＿＿＿＿＿＿＿＿＿＿＿＿＿＿＿＿＿＿＿＿＿＿＿＿

＿＿＿＿＿＿＿＿＿＿＿＿＿＿＿＿＿＿＿＿＿＿＿＿

＿＿＿＿＿＿＿＿＿＿＿＿＿＿＿＿＿＿＿＿＿＿＿＿

＿＿＿＿＿＿＿＿＿＿＿＿＿＿＿＿＿＿＿＿＿＿＿＿

＿＿＿＿＿＿＿＿＿＿＿＿＿＿＿＿＿＿＿＿＿＿＿＿

Short-term Goal(s)＿＿＿＿＿＿＿＿ Rewards ＿＿＿＿＿＿＿

Make an appointment with physician/nutritionist.

＿＿＿＿＿＿＿＿＿＿＿＿＿＿＿＿＿＿＿＿＿＿＿＿

＿＿＿＿＿＿＿＿＿＿＿＿＿＿＿＿＿＿＿＿＿＿＿＿

＿＿＿＿＿＿＿＿＿＿＿＿＿＿＿＿＿＿＿＿＿＿＿＿

＿＿＿＿＿＿＿＿＿＿＿＿＿＿＿＿＿＿＿＿＿＿＿＿

＿＿＿＿＿＿＿＿＿＿＿＿＿＿＿＿＿＿＿＿＿＿＿＿

＿＿＿＿＿＿＿＿＿＿＿＿＿＿＿＿＿＿＿＿＿＿＿＿

＿＿＿＿＿＿＿＿＿＿＿＿＿＿＿＿＿＿＿＿＿＿＿＿

Reminder Notes: ＿＿＿＿＿＿＿＿＿＿＿＿＿＿＿＿＿

＿＿＿＿＿＿＿＿＿＿＿＿＿＿＿＿＿＿＿＿＿＿＿＿

＿＿＿＿＿＿＿＿＿＿＿＿＿＿＿＿＿＿＿＿＿＿＿＿

＿＿＿＿＿＿＿＿＿＿＿＿＿＿＿＿＿＿＿＿＿＿＿＿

＿＿＿＿＿＿＿＿＿＿＿＿＿＿＿＿＿＿＿＿＿＿＿＿

＿＿＿＿＿＿＿＿＿＿＿＿＿＿＿＿＿＿＿＿＿＿＿＿

NOTES

The Latest Research On Minerals And Other Important Supplements

What About Mineral Supplements?*

In addition to the vitamins discussed in chapter 14, there are four minerals that the body uses to ward off stress. These are calcium, potassium, magnesium and zinc.

Besides the four antistress minerals which will be discussed in the section below, there are some other important supplements which have been recognized as essential parts of a good nutrition program. You will want to discuss any possible supplement program with your nutritionist.

*WARNING: Do not take mineral supplements without the approval of your physician or nutritionist.

What About Calcium?

Calcium could be called the muscle and bone mineral because of its important role in the formation and maintenance of bones and in the contraction of the muscles. Calcium is also essential to the blood-clotting process, to maintaining a steady heartbeat and to nerve transmission.

Positive Checklist for Calcium

Solubility: Acid   **Min. Daily Req.: 800 to 1200 mg.**

---

* Essential to bone formation

* Promotes good teeth

* Promotes proper blood clotting

* Maintains proper heartbeat

* Essential for muscle activity

* Protects against the effects of
    radioactive strontium 90

* Speeds up the healing process

* Essential for the use of vitamins A, C, D

Calcium can be obtained from a wide variety of animal and vegetarian sources. As part of the effort to eliminate fat and reduce cholesterol, preference would be to rely on vegetarian sources wherever possible.

Natural Food Sources of Calcium

Vegetarian	Animal*
Almonds	*Lacto/Ovo*
Blackstrap molasses	Milk
Broccoli	Cheese
Brussel sprouts	Yogurt
Cabbage	

Natural Food Sources of Calcium

Vegetarian	Animal*
Carrots	Eggs
Dandelion greens	
Collards	
Endive	
Grapefruit	
Kale	*Meat/Fish*
Millet	Clams
Navy beans	Oysters
Oats	Salmon
Parsley	Sardines
Raw vegetables	Liver
Romaine lettuce	
Sesame seeds	
Spinach	
Sunflower seeds	
Soybeans	
Tortillas	
Turnip greens	
Walnuts	
Watercress	

*Note: Milk and milk products are the richest sources of calcium. Strict vegetarians may want to consider supplements.

There is increasing evidence that calcium excretion is promoted by a high-protein diet. With age, the body is less able to absorb calcium. According to some researchers, calcium deficiencies are more widespread in the general population than you would think. Early signs of deficiency are foot and leg cramps and insomnia.

Facts About Calcium

Symptoms of Deficiency	Symptoms of Overdose	Things That Use The Vitamin Up Too Fast
Heart palpitations	Toxic dose not	Stress
Insomnia	reported.	No exercise
Muscle cramps		Too much
Grogginess		saturated fat

Facts About Calcium
continued

Symptoms of Deficiency	Symptoms of Overdose	Things That Use The Vitamin Up Too Fast
Nervousness	Toxic dose not reported.	Stress
Depression		No exercise
Porous bones		Too much saturated fat
Rickets		
Tooth decay		
Irritability		
Brittle nails		

Calcium should be taken along with magnesium. The usual ratio is two parts calcium to one part magnesium. Approximately 70% to 80% of calcium is excreted by the body. It is very important for pregnant and breast-feeding women to have a sufficient calcium intake. About 90% of the calcium in the body is in the bones. According to many nutrition experts, the body replaces all the calcium every six years. If you are not getting enough calcium from the food you eat, it is withdrawn from the bones and teeth. Remember, mineral supplements should be taken along with vitamin supplements in a balanced formula.

What About Potassium?

Potassium could be called the anti-acid mineral because of its important role in the maintenance of the acid-alkaline balance of the blood. It also plays an important role in helping your heart maintain its proper beat.

Positive Checklist for Potassium

Solubility: Water   Min. Daily Req.: 2000 to 2500 mg.

* Prevents low blood sugar

* Promotes a steady heartbeat

* Essential for good muscle contraction

* Promotes hormone secretions

* Prevents female disorders

* Promotes proper acid-alkaline balance

Potassium can be obtained from a wide variety of animal and vegetarian sources. As part of the effort to eliminate fat and reduce cholesterol, the preference would be to rely on vegetarian sources.

Natural Food Sources of Potassium

Vegetarian	Animal
Apricots	*Lacto/Ovo:*
Bananas	Milk
Blackstrap molasses	Yogurt
Dates	
Green leafy vegetables	
Nuts	
Oranges	
Peaches	
Peanuts	
Potatoes	
Raisins	*Meat/Fish*
Sunflower seeds	Seafood
Whole grains	

Too much sugar can result in a potassium deficiency. Since potassium is essential to the metabolism of sugar and the formation of glycogen, a deficiency of potassium can result in **low blood sugar.**

Facts About Potassium

Symptoms of Deficiency	Symptoms of Overdose	Things That Use The Vitamin Up Too Fast
Acne	Toxic dose not reported.	Stress
Insomnia		Alcohol
Muscle weakness		Coffee
Dry skin		Salt
Nervousness		Sugar
Excessive salt retention		Aspirin
Continuous thirst		Laxatives
Constipation		Diuretics
Muscle damage		Steroids
Extreme fatigue		
Low blood sugar		
Slow and irregular heartbeat		
Weak reflexes		
High blood pressure		

Potassium intake should be about the same as your salt intake. Your exact potassium needs may be different from everyone else's and are related to the amount of salt you use. Potassium is an important part of the mineral base of your muscles and helps to make them flexible. Approximately 90% of your potassium intake is excreted in the urine. Remember, mineral supplements should be taken along with vitamin supplements in a balanced formula.

What About Magnesium?

Magnesium could be called the natural tranquilizer mineral because of its important role in the nervous system. Chemical fertilizers cause food to be deficient in magnesium. Boiling or soaking food causes a loss of magnesium.

Positive Checklist for Magnesium

Solubility: Water   **Min. Daily Req.: 350 mg. for males**
300 mg. for females

* Essential for a healthy heart

* Helps body retain calcium

* Helps body retain potassium

* Helps body use fats and starches

* Helps regulate blood sugar

* Makes teeth and bones harder

* Helps build strong lung tissue

* Helps body use vitamins C, E, B1

Magnesium can be obtained from a wide variety of animal and vegetarian sources. As part of the effort to eliminate fat and reduce cholesterol, the preference would be to rely on vegetarian sources.

Natural Food Sources of Magnesium

Vegetarian	Animal
Alfalfa	*Meat/Fish*
Almonds	Seafood
Apples	
Bran	
Beet greens	
Brown rice	
Cashews	
Celery	
Chard	
Dates	
Endive	
Figs	
Green veggies	
Honey	
Kale	
Lemons	
Lima beans	
Nuts	
Oatmeal	
Peanuts	
Peaches	
Raisins	
Sesame seeds	
Spinach	
Soybeans	
Sunflower seeds	
Whole grains	

In addition to helping your body maintain the desired acid-alkaline balance, magnesium helps your body use vitamin C and calcium, essential elements in the prevention of stress symptoms. Magnesium is necessary for proper functioning of muscles and nerves. Since every cell in your body needs magnesium to function properly, a deficiency could cause you to have severe physical and/or mental problems. In addition, a deficiency of magnesium leads to deficiencies of calcium and potassium. This can lead to kidney damage, kidney stones and heart attack.

Facts About Magnesium

Symptoms of Deficiency*	Symptoms of Overdose	Things That Use The Vitamin Up Too Fast
Rapid pulse	Toxic dose	Alcohol
Insomnia	30,000 mg.	Excess calcium
		Too much
Confusion		saturated fat
Restlessness		Vomiting
Mental disorientation		Diarrhea
Tremors		
Seizures		
Premature wrinkles		
Kidney stones		
Muscle cramps		
Heart attack		

*Note: Magnesium deficiency can cause loss of calcium and potassium, giving you their deficiency symptoms also.

Only about 30% to 40% of the magnesium that you take in with your food is absorbed. The rest is excreted in both your urine and feces, with the majority being excreted in your urine. There is some evidence that magnesium plays a role in the prevention of cardiovascular disease. Remember, mineral supplements should be taken along with vitamin supplements in a balanced formula.

What About Zinc?

Zinc could be called the healing mineral because of its important role in healing wounds and burns. Zinc is required to form the insulin molecule and is therefore involved in carbohydrate and energy metabolism.

Positive Checklist for Zinc

Solubility: Acid   **Min. Daily Req.: 15 mg.**

---

* Essential to bone formation

* Promotes good teeth

* Promotes proper blood clotting

* Maintains proper heartbeat

* Essential for muscle activity

* Protects against the effects of radioactive strontium 90

* Speeds up healing process

* Essential for use of vitamins A, C, D

Zinc is a trace mineral which is found in decreasing amounts in our soil and therefore in our plants, due to the use of chemical fertilizers. It is available in a variety of animal and vegetarian sources. As part of the effort to eliminate fat and reduce cholesterol, the preference would be to rely on vegetarian sources.

Natural Food Sources of Zinc

Vegetarian	Animal
Brewer's yeast	*Lacto/Ovo*
Green leafy veggies	Milk
Mushrooms	Eggs
Onions	
Nuts	
Soybeans	*Meat/Fish*
Spinach	Liver
Sunflower seeds	Oysters
Wheat bran	Herring
Wheat germ	

A deficiency of zinc can lead to various reproductive-organ problems, from delayed sexual maturity, to enlarged prostate glands to sterility. Early signs of zinc deficiency are white spots on fingernails and toenails.

Facts About Zinc

Symptoms of Deficiency	Symptoms of Overdose	Things That Use The Vitamin Up Too Fast
White spots on nails	Toxic dose not reported.	Alcohol
Sterility		Oral contraceptives
Delayed sexual maturity		Too much calcium
Fatigue		
Wounds heal slowly		
Burns heal slowly		
Enlarged prostate		
Hair loss		
Lowered sex drive		
Anorexia		
Diminished taste and smell		
Dandruff		
Low resistance to infection		

Zinc reserves in your body are not easily harnessed, which means that there is a need for an ongoing, regular ingestion of zinc. This is particularly important during times of stress or periods of growth.

Remember, mineral supplements should be taken along with vitamin supplements in a balanced formula.

WHAT ARE SOME OF THE OTHER IMPORTANT SUPPLEMENTS?

In addition to the antistress vitamins and minerals, there are a number of other important supplements you may want to consider. Among the more important ones are the fat-soluble vitamins A, D and E, and the minerals iron and selenium. All are important to good nutrition and to protecting yourself from the environment. Besides the vitamins and minerals listed in the chart below, there are other supplements that you may want to explore with your nutritionist.

Summary Checklist for Some Important Supplements

Supplement	What It Does For You	Recommended Daily Allowance
Vitamin A	* Helps resist infection * Helps night vision * Retards aging process * Keeps testicles healthy * Prevents eye diseases * Nourishes skin and hair	4800 to 6000 IU*

Summary Checklist For Some Important Supplements, continued

Supplement	What It Does For You	Recommended Daily Allowance
Vitamin D	* Promotes bone formation * Prevents tooth decay * Prevents gum disease * Prevents rickets * Keeps thyroid healthy	200 to 400 IU*
Vitamin E	* Retards aging process * Prevents scar-tissue formation * Prevents blood clots * Promotes healthy sex organs * Promotes male potency	15 IU
Iron	* Prevents anemia * Helps you fight stress * Promotes growth in children * Builds up your blood	10 mg. for males 18 mg. for females
Selenium	* Powerful antioxidant against air, water, food pollution * Prevents red blood cell damage * May slow down aging * Reduces risk of cancer	Not established.*

*WARNING: Overdoses can be dangerous to your health. Do not take supplements without the approval of your physician or nutritionist.

CHAPTER FIFTEEN WORKSHEET

Long-term Goal(s)   Rewards

Determine supplemental needs _____

_____

_____

_____

_____

_____

_____

_____

_____

Short-term Goals   Rewards

_____

_____

_____

_____

_____

_____

_____

_____

_____

_____

_____

Reminder Notes: _____

Make appointment with physician/nutritionist _____

_____

_____

CHAPTER SIXTEEN

Can Supplements Heal And Protect Me?

Can Supplements Protect Me?*

One of the saddest facts of our industrialized society is that our food, water, soil and air are full of toxic chemicals. Food supplements are increasingly being recognized as successful ways to counteract the effects of the poisons in our environment.

The chart below will give you an idea of how food supplements can be used to protect you from the harmful effects of the poisons in your environment.

*WARNING: Do not take food supplements without the approval of your physician or nutritionist.

Protective Properties of Specific Foods And Supplements*

Supplement/Food	What Does It Protect Against?
Algin	Lead, strontium 90
Brewer's yeast	Mercury, strontium 90, X-rays
Buttermilk	DDT, toxic drugs
Calcium	Lead, mercury, strontium 90
Kelp	Strontium 90, radioactive iodine

Protective Properties of Specific Food Supplements* (Continued)

Supplement	What Does It Protect Against?
Lecithin	Lead, mercury, DDT, strontium 90, X-rays, toxic drugs, nitrates, nitrites
Magnesium	Strontium 90
Pectin	Strontium 90
Yogurt	DDT, toxic drugs
Zinc	Cadmium
Vitamin A	Carbon monoxide, lead, nitrates
Vitamin C	Lead, DDT, cadmium, strontium 90, X-rays, toxic drugs, nitrates
Vitamin D	Lead
Vitamin E	Carbon monoxide, lead, strontium 90, toxic drugs, nitrates
Vitamin F	X-rays
Vitamin P (Bioflavonoids)	Exzema, hypertension, rheumatism, ulcers
Vitamin B-Complex	Lead, strontium 90, toxic drugs
Vitamin B1	Lead
Vitamin B5 (pantothenic acid)	X-rays
Inositol (B-complex)	X-rays

*Note: Consult your nutritionist for amounts to take.

Can Supplements Help Me With My Problem?

You should consult your physician and nutritionist about the possibility of using vitamin therapy. The chart on the next page will give you an idea of some of the ways supplements have been successfully used to treat various medical and psychological problems.

Therapeutic Applications Of Supplements*

Conditions Treated	Supplements Used
Acne	A, B2, niacin, D, potassium
Alcoholism	A, B1, B2, B12, C, D, choline, folic acid, iron, magnesium, zinc, potassium
Allergies	A, B2, C, D, E, potassium, pantothenic acid
Anemia	B1, B12, folic acid, iron
Arthritis	A, B1, B2, B12, niacin, pantothenic acid, C, D, E, calcium
Asthma	A, biotin, B12
Atherosclerosis	B6, choline, inositol, C, E, zinc, folic acid
Athlete's foot	B2
Aging symptoms	B1, calcium, E, pantothenic acid
Baldness	B2, biotin, choline, folic acid, inositol, niacin, pantothenic acid, PABA, copper, zinc
Bronchitis	A, biotin
Bursitis	B12
Burns	Potassium, E, zinc

Therapeutic Applications Of Supplements

Conditions Treated	Supplements Used
Bruising	K
Cholesterol (high)	A, B6, C, E, F, P, magnesium, zinc, choline, inositol
Constipation	B-complex, B1, choline, inositol
Circulatory problems	Folic acid, choline, niacin, potassium
Colds	A, C
Cramps (muscles, legs, etc.)	Biotin, niacin, calcium
Depression	Biotin, magnesium
Diabetes	A, B1, B2, E, chromium, potassium, zinc
Diarrhea	B1, B2, niacin
Digestive problems	B1, B2, pantothenic acid, iron, magnesium
Eczema	A, B6, biotin, D, F, P, PABA
Fatigue	B-complex, B12, folic acid, pantothenic acid

Therapeutic Applications Of Supplements, continued

Conditions Treated	Supplements Used
Gray hair	PABA
Heart disease/problems	A, B-complex, B1, C, E, F, choline, inositol, potassium, magnesium
Hypoglycemia	B-complex, B6, B12, C, choline, chromium, pantothenic acid
Headaches (including migranes)	A, B-complex, B6, E, calcium, choline, niacin
Healing	E, zinc
Insomnia	B12, calcium, choline
Menopause	Calcium, E
Menstrual problems	B-complex, B6, E, K, calcium, folic acid
Nervousness	B-complex, calcium, iron, magnesium
Prostate problems	Zinc, iron
Rheumatism	P, calcium
Stress	B-complex, B1, B2, B6, B12, C, D, folic acid, niacin, PABA, pantothenic acid
Tooth decay	A, C, niacin, magnesium, pantothenic acid, phosphorus
Ulcers	P, folic acid

Note: Consult your nutritionist for amounts to take.

CHAPTER SIXTEEN WORKSHEET

Long-term Goal(s)_____ Rewards_____

Determine supplemental needs

_____

_____

_____

_____

_____

_____

Short-term Goals _____Rewards _____

Make appointment with physician

_____

_____

_____

_____

_____

_____

Reminder Notes: _____

_____

_____

_____

_____

CHAPTER SEVENTEEN
Fasting For
Healthy Living

America is a land of boundless natural
resources and rich, fertile land. This land
has given Americans one of the highest
standards of living in the world. Unfortunately, our land of plenty has become a
double-edged sword.

Many Americans do not get the proper
nutrients in their diet because they eat
too much of the wrong foods! In addition,
our food, water and air have been contaminated by the by-products of the very
processes that have given us our material
wealth. The end result is that most
chronic diseases are related to our own
overindulgence in food and drink or to
contaminated food, air and water.

Is there a way to cleanse our bodies of all
these toxins, to rejuvenate the cells, to
reduce the incidence of chronic diseases
and extend the number of healthy years
that we have here on earth? Some experts
claim that periodic fasting followed by
proper nutrition is the answer.

What Is This Chapter About?

This chapter will teach you the benefits of
fasting and the types of fasting, and introduce you to the most widely accepted

methods of fasting. **WARNING: Do not fast without your physician's approval and without having had a complete physical examination.** We are not physicians nor are we nutritionists. The information in this chapter is not prescriptive but is presented for your education. While most experts on fasting say that a person who is not suffering from a major disease such as cancer, diabetes or heart disease can fast safely for up to three days without supervision, we recommend that you get the approval of your physician before you try it.

Fasting Throughout History

Fasting as a means of purifying the body and lifting the spirit has been a way of life for those practicing yoga for 10,000 years or more. It has its roots in religious and mystical tribal rites among the American Indians, Hindus, and ancient Hebrews and Greeks. Moses, Elijah and Jesus fasted. In modern times, both Christians, Jews and Muslims celebrate certain religious periods with brief fasting. In ancient times, people were often faced with days, even weeks, of little or no food due to natural disasters, poor weather, etc. Going without food, deliberately or involuntarily, has been part of our evolutionary history.

In recent years there has been increased interest in fasting to clean the body of toxins and help rejuvenate body tissues and cells long abused by improper dietary habits. Simultaneously, scientists have been studying the effects of restricted caloric diets and fasting on increasing the life span.

What Does Science Say About Fasting?

Fasting is used to rejuvenate and to cure specific medical problems in other parts of the world; however, the practice is not generally accepted in the United States.

We did several comprehensive computer searches at a major university library on the topics of fasting, health and aging. We found a sparsity of research literature on fasting with human beings. We did find research with rats and other animals on prolonging life through fasting. The evidence presented in this research is overwhelmingly clear. When animals are put on a restricted caloric intake which includes fasting, the fasted animals outlive the normally fed animals. The earlier studies found that life extension through fasting worked only when begun with very young rats. Later research suggests that you can begin later in maturity and still extend your life span through fasting. Please note that good nutrition during non-fasting conditions is essential!

What Can Fasting Do For Me?*

1. **PHYSICAL BENEFITS**
   * Abnormal cells used up
   * Organs given a rest
   * Healing process speeded up
   * Food assimilation improved
   * Waste-elimination system improved
   * Immune system rejuvenated
   * Tissues Rejuvenated

2. **PSYCHOLOGICAL BENEFITS**
   * You feel lighter
   * Your mind seems to work better
   * You look younger and your self-concept is improved

*Note: Benefits were taken from individual clinical reports and case studies and/or scientifically controlled research data on animals.

WARNING: We do not recommend that you fast in order to lose weight. See your physician or nutritionist for help in establishing an individualized permanent weight loss nutritional program.

Will Fasting Extend My Life?

No one knows for certain. However, there are numerous studies that show that the life span of rats can be increased by as much as 40% by restricting their calories. One of the methods of restricting calories is periodic fasting followed by periods of systematic undereating of highly nutritious foods and supplements.

Dr. Roy Walford, a physician who has devoted much of his professional research to studying the causes of aging, is a well-known advocate of fasting as part of a program of restricted caloric intake. His approach to life extension appears to be based largely on studies made with rats. This same approach for maintaining vibrant health has been advocated for years by Dr. Paavo Airola, a best-selling author of books on maintaining good health through proper nutrition and diet. Most of his recommendations appear to be based on studies done in Europe and other parts of the world.

What Happens When You Fast?

---

1. **YOUR BODY USES UP ABNORMAL CELLS** According to the experts on both juice and water fasting, the primary benefit of fasting is its ability to rid your body of damaged and diseased tissues and cells through a process of self-digestion called autolysis. During fasting, the body lives off itself by

using up inferior materials such as tumors and dead cells. This process may explain some of the reported cures. It is the beginning of what many proponents call the rejuvenation process.

2. **YOUR BODY BUILDS NEW CELLS**

According to the experts, another advantage of fasting is that your body is stimulated to build new and healthy cells and tissues. In studies with rats who were kept on restricted nutritional programs, they were found to be chemically younger than the control-group rats on a number of biochemical indices (e.g., blood cholesterol levels of older fasted rats were those of much younger rats).

3. **YOUR BODY ELIMINATES TOXINS AND WASTE**

Since your body does not have to concern itself with digestion, it uses this period to burn up old inferior cells and build new and healthier ones. It also begins to eliminate the accumulation of toxins in the body. The total process of burning up inferior tissues, eliminating waste and toxins and building up new cells adds up to a form of self-rejuvenation.

4. **YOUR ENTIRE SYSTEM IS ABLE TO REST**

Another advantage of fasting is that it gives your entire digestive system and other related organs a rest. After fasting, according to the experts, your body functions more efficiently. Part of this is attributed to the self-imposed rest of fasting.

5. **YOUR RISK OF DISEASE IS LOWERED**

In studies with rodents and pigeons on restricted diets, the risks of getting cancer, kidney disease, heart disease, vascular disease and arteriosclerosis were reduced dramatically. In one study, the incidence of breast cancer was reduced in some strains of mice practically to zero.

6. **YOUR IMMUNE SYSTEM IS REJUVENATED**

In the normal pattern of aging, your immune system becomes inefficient. As you age, it gradually loses its ability to tell the difference between cells in your body that are "you" and cells that don't belong there (i.e., germs). When this happens, there can be active self-destruction! With time and nutritional abuse, the immune system gets worn out and loses much of its ability to repair damage and handle toxic materials. Research has shown that the immune system can be rejuvenated by periodic fasting alternated with good nutrition.

7. **YOUR CHANCES OF LIVING A LONGER LIFE ARE INCREASED**

A series of experiments with rodents and other animals has shown that life spans can be increased as much as 40% by sharply curtailing the number of calories in the diet. On a restricted calorie diet, only the total number of calories per week is limited but critical nutrients are not! Long before modern science got into the act, yoga practitioners advocated systematic control of foods and routine fasting as a method of prolonging youthfulness of the body. They were only 10,000 years ahead of our rat scientists!

There are purists who say that eating nothing and drinking only pure water is the only true fasting. Then there are those who say that drinking only freshly made juice while eating nothing is also fasting. The chart below describes the approaches in more detail. Please note that no matter which method you read about, the advocates claim the same benefits as those listed in the preceding chart.

1. **WATER-ONLY FAST**   This is the traditional way of fasting. Proponents of this method drink only pure water during the fast. They believe you must not be very physically or socially active during this period. Fasting takes place in a calm environment, and during this period of time you should not take hot baths or enemas.

2. **JUICE-ONLY FAST**   The advocates of juice-fasting say that it is safer than water-fasting because all of the essential nutrients are supplied to your bloodstream from juices and broths. They claim this approach gives you all the advantages of water-fasting without the possible loss of precious nutrients. During a juice fast, most advocates recommend a combination of fresh fruit and/or vegetable juices. You are usually allowed to perform some light physical activity and drink certain herb teas, and are instructed to take one or two enemas a day. The rationale for enemas is that they will help your body eliminate poisons that are left in your colon from the chemical processes associated with fasting.

3. **MONO-FAST**   Mono-fasts are simply a way of giving your body a rest from the digestive process without giving up eating. The practice is to choose one food and eat only that food for the fasting period. Commonly used in mono-fasts are beets, carrots, apples, brown rice, millet, rye, corn or barley. Mono-fasts are frequently recommended in place of the other two fasting methods for the winter season in cold climates because the body stays warmer. Proponents of mono-fasting claim results similar to those of the other methods.

How Do I Learn To Fast?

1. First, before you go any farther with the idea of fasting, you must get a physical checkup and the approval of your physician.

2. For first-time fasters, we recommend that you get professional guidance from a health practitioner who has supervised fasts for therapeutic and/or rejuvenation purposes. The first time we fasted, we did just that. If anything, the monitoring helped take away any doubts we had about the process.

According to the experts, most people can fast for a week to ten days quite safely. There are a number of fasting spas in which you can enroll. This is probably the best way for first-time fasters who plan an extensive fast.

3. Assuming you intend to fast for a short time and the results of your physical examination permit you to try it, remember that the experts say that fasting is perfectly safe for almost anyone if (1) you follow the accepted rules of beginning and breaking a fast and (2) your fast does not last more than a week.

4. Last, you must prepare yourself psychologically for the fast. The chart below outlines the steps you should follow to fast successfully.

Nine Steps to Successful Fasting

A Psychological Approach

1. PREPARE YOURSELF MENTALLY

Learn everything you can about fasting before you make a decision to fast. If you have any doubts, do not fast. You must have an optimistic attitude or you will fail dismally. Plan a short fast so that you can have some success. We recommend that you do a mono-fast for one day for your first try. We did an apple fast our first time. If you will pardon the expression, it was a piece of cake! Every time we got hungry we ate a nice, fresh apple! A week later we did a one-day juice fast.

Motivate yourself. Make it a point to read several books on fasting. Most of them contain case studies of people who have been remarkably rejuvenated by fasting. These stories can help you become motivated to stick with it.

Learn what to expect. Knowledge of what to expect when you fast can defuse any fears or doubts that you have. Many of the case studies and books on fasting describe in detail exactly how your body will react during a fast. Remember, fasting is not starving. You are not starving until your body begins to feed on vital tissues. According to the experts, this does not occur until about 30 days into a fast, at which time your appetite will return. Remember, also, that you will not be hungry after the third day of a fast. Your appetite will go away naturally as your body begins to feed on its defective and unwanted tissues.

2. PREPARE YOURSELF SOCIALLY

Whatever your personal household arrangements, you must do some advance work. You need to "advertise" to those around you what you plan to do and when. Try to enlist their help and support. It will make it easier if you deal with any objections from those around you before you fast. Make it quite clear, however, that you intend to go through with the fast with or without their approval and that you expect them to respect your rights! Any attempt by them to take you away from your goals should be dealt with directly. Anyone who tries these tactics cannot have much respect for you and should be dealt with accordingly.

The best way is to team-fast. We fast together. That way we eliminate the smell of food in the house and have each other for moral support. As you become more experienced at fasting, it becomes easier. Now that we are experienced, short-term fasters, we can actually sit at a dinner table and watch people eat when we are fasting.

3. PREPARE YOURSELF NUTRITIONALLY AND PHYSICALLY

If you are planning a fast of more than a couple of days, eat very lightly for one to three days preceding the fast. Eat raw or lightly steamed vegetables. Plain brown rice is okay.

If the fast is to last for more than three days, most experts on fasting recommend that you take a purgative the night before you begin the fast. Consult your health practitioner on which one to take. Health-food stores sell herbal laxatives that are supposed to do the trick with a minimum of irritation to your system. If you are only going to fast one day, purgatives are not necessary.

The major drawback to fasting for most people who try it for the first time is the issue of enemas. The arguments for and against enemas both make sense.

On the pro side, fasting experts claim that since you are not eating, the bowel action (peristalsis) is not stimulated, with the result that accumulated toxins released by the fasting process will re-enter the bloodstream through the colon wall. They argue that enemas will make certain that you excrete these poisons.

Equally convincing is the argument against enemas by other fasting experts. They claim that the body will naturally expel unwanted toxins as needed and that enemas will rob your intestinal tract of valuable bacteria.

If you are only going to fast for one to three days, you don't really need to take enemas.

If your juice or water fast is to be longer than 3 days, consult your physician about the advisability of taking enemas. When we fast more than two days at a time, we usually take enemas because several of the medical and naturopathic experts on fasting make a strong case for doing so.

4. **PLAN ACTIVITIES THAT KEEP YOUR MIND OFF FOOD**

You won't want to do strenuous exercise, but bed rest isn't essential either. We usually take long walks, short shopping trips, watch video movies, catch up on our social correspondence, read books for pleasure that we've been putting aside for just such an occasion, etc. For very short one-day fasts, just carry on your everyday activities minus the meals! Sunbaths are also very good for you!

5. **PLAN FOR MENTAL HEALING EXERCISES**

Increase your meditation to two or three times per day. Create visualization exercises (see Chapter 7) that help you get the most out of the physical process of fasting. See your self getting younger as a result of the fasting process. Visualize your body ridding itself of defective tissues and cells, eliminating toxins that have built up, etc.

6. **CONTROL YOUR ENVIRONMENT**

Put yourself in a place where you will be free of the temptation to break the fast. This is particularly important for the first three days of a fast. After that, your appetite will disappear naturally.

7. **CONTROL THE QUALITY OF THE LIQUIDS YOU DRINK WHILE FASTING**

Do not drink stimulants such as coffee, regular tea, alcohol, etc. You can drink a modest amount of herb teas like peppermint, rose hips and chamomile, but stay away from coffee substitutes. One of our favorites is pure hot water with freshly squeezed lemon juice. (Don't overdo this because of the acid.)

Drink only pure water from your well, bottled spring water or distilled water.

If you are juice-fasting, drink only **freshly squeezed vegetable or fruit juices.** We use only carrot, apple or pear juice. Get a good electric juicer. Don't make the juice up ahead of time because it oxidizes rather quickly. If you have to go to work, it's okay to make up a little to take with you if you have a way to keep it cool.

| 8. | **BREAK YOUR FAST SLOWLY** | Every expert on fasting emphasizes this point. If you want to reap the benefits of your fast, you must break the fast slowly. Eat slowly, chew your food and **don't overeat.** Get back to eating gradually by introducing one food at a time into your diet. Begin with fruit or a salad and gradually add heavier food. Continue to avoid stimulants. |

| 9. | **REWARD YOURSELF** | As we have mentioned on many occasions in this text, people repeat behaviors that are rewarded and stop behaviors that are not rewarded. Make sure that during the course of the fast you have non-food rewards that you give yourself. Have a special reward when you have successfully broken the fast. One of our favorite series of rewards is the time to do something we want to do, such as reading a novel. A good reward for some people is a new pair of slacks or other article of clothing that goes with your new image of youthfulness. |

The Choice Is Yours

In summary, the literature is full of articles and books on various methods of fasting, most of it is based on individual case studies. Part of the reason for this condition is lack of interest in a subject that many medical practitioners consider to be "quackery." The other reason is that it is very difficult to run controlled fasting experiments with human beings. At any rate, the case study data on humans who fast properly suggests that there are many benefits to the process for most people.

In terms of scientific controlled experiments, the research has been done primarily with animals, mostly with rats. The results speak for themselves: fasted rats who receive essential nutrients have dramatically increased life spans when compared to control group rats fed normally. They also have dramatically lower incidences of such illnesses as cancer and heart disease. And using a number of biochemical tests, they are younger chemically. Anyone with a logical mind would ask the question: "Can we assume that because it works with rats, it will work with humans?" There is no final answer to that question, but we fast.

CHAPTER SEVENTEEN WORKSHEET

Long-term Goal(s)   Rewards
Determine fasting needs.

_____

_____

_____

Short-term Goal(s)   Rewards
Make appointment with physician.

_____

_____

Reminder Notes: _____

_____

_____

_____

EPILOGUE

The book has presented you with a 3% formula for staying young, healthy and sexy. It works—but only if you make it work! Our final words of advice are these:

START TODAY

Even if you do only one little thing today, one little thing is better than nothing.

DO IT FOR YOURSELF

Don't do this for your spouse, your children, your business or for any other reason. Do it for yourself! You've been taking care of other people all of your life. Now it's time to take care of you!

DON'T EXPECT TO BE PERFECT

When you fall off the wagon, as you will, don't consider yourself a failure. Consider yourself human. Progress is never in a straight line. It's a series of zigzags and plateaus. The real mark of a winner is the ability to pick yourself up, dust yourself off, and keep going.

EXPECT TO SUCCEED

You can do it!

REFERENCES

Abehsera, Michel, **Zen Macrobiotic Cooking**, New York, New York: Avon Books, 1968.

Adams, Ruth and Murray, Frank, **Megavitamin Therapy**, New York, New York: Larchmont Books, 1973.

Airola, Paavo, **Are You Confused**, Phoenix, Arizona: Health Plus Publishers, 1971.

Airola, Paavo, **How to Get Well**, Phoenix, Arizona: Health Plus Publishers, 1974.

Airola, Paavo, **How to Keep Slim, Healthy and Young with Juice Fasting**, Phoenix, Arizona: Health Plus Publishers, 1971.

Airola, Paavo, **Hypoglycemia: A Better Approach**, Phoenix, Arizona: Health Plus Publishers, 1977.

Airola, Paavo, **The Miracle of Garlic**, Phoenix, Arizona: Health Plus Publishers, 1978.

Airola, Paavo, **There Is a Cure for Arthritis**, West Nyack, New York: Parker Publishing Company, Inc., 1968.

Akers, Keith, Why people get fat, **Vegetarian Times**, May 1983, 28- 31.

Alberti, Robert E. and Emmons, Michael L., **Stand Up, Speak Out, Talk Back**, New York, New York: Pocket Books, 1975.

Alcantara, E. N. and Speckmann, E. W., Diet, nutrition, and cancer, **American Journal of Clinical Nutrition**, 1976, Vol. 29, 1035-1047.

Alderman, M. H., Communities with unusally short life-spans: the effects of life-style modification, **Bulletin of the New York Academy of Medicine**, March 1979, 55(3), 357-366.

Alexander, F. M., **The Use of the Self**, Downey, California: Centerline Press, April 1984.

An after-dinner walk speeds weight loss, **Prevention**, April 1984, pp. 96.

Anderson, T. W., Reid, D. B. and Beaton, G. H., Vitamin C and serum-cholesterol, **Lancet**, October 1972, 2(782), 876-877.

Anderson, T. W., Reid, D. B. and Beaton, G. H., Vitamin C and the common cold: a double-blind trial, **Canadian Medical Association Journal**, September 1972, 107(6), 503-508.

Anderson, T. W., Suranyi, G. and Beaton, G. H., The effect on winter illness of large doses of vitamin C, **Canadian Medical Association Journal,** July 1974, 111(1), 31-36.

Angrist, B. and Gershon, S., Clinical effects of amphetamine and L-Dopa on sexuality and aggression, **Comprehensive Psychiatry**, June, 1976, Vol. 17, 715-722.

Arehart-Treichel, J., Can your personality kill you?, **New York Magazine**, November 1977, 10:62-67.

Armstrong, D. E., Performance as a function of expressed and nonexpressed levels of aspiration, Unpublished masters thesis, Howard University, 1947.

Arrangio, J., The effects of individual goal-setting conferences and classrooms instruction in human relations on locus of control, school attendance and alienation of disadvantaged high school students, Unpublished doctoral dissertation, Boston Univeristy, 1980.

Bandura, Albert and Adams, Nancy E., Analysis of self-efficacy theory of behavioral change, **Cognitive Therapy & Research.** December 1977, 1(4), 287-310.

Bandura, Albert, Blanchard, Edward B. and Ritter, Brunhilde, Relative efficacy of desensitization and modeling approaches for inducing behavioral, affective, and attitudinal changes. **Journal of Personality & Social Psychology**, 1969, 13(3), 173- 199.

Bandura, Albert, **Social Learning Theory**, Englewood Cliffs, New Jersey: Prentice-Hall, Inc., 1977.

Barker, Sarah, **The Alexander Technique**, New York, New York: Bantam Books, 1978.

Barlow, Wilfred, **The Alexander Technique**, New York, New York: Warner Books, 1973.

Barrows, C. H., Kokkonen, G. C., Genetic information and the life-span of laboratory animal models, **Review of Pure Applications of Pharmacological Science**, Oct.-Dec. 1980, 1(4), 293-325.

Bartus, R. T., Four stimulants of the central nervous system: effects on short-term memory in young versus aged monkeys, **Journal of the American Geriatrics Society**, July 1979, 27(7), 289-297.

Batten, Joe, **Expectations and Possibilities**, Reading, Massachusetts: Addison-Wesley Publishing Company, 1981.

Beatty, G. J. & Gardner, D. C., Goal setting and resume writing as a locus of control change technique with college women, **College Student Journal**, 13(1):315-318, 1979.

Bechtel, Stefan, Nutrients that help your body heal itself, **Prevention**, August 1982, 89-90, 92-93.

Bechtel, Stephan, Vitamin C: Changing your body for the better, **Prevention**, September 1982, 20, 22-24, 26.

Beck, S. D. and Bharadwaj, R. K., Reversed development and cellular aging in an insect, **Science**, 1972, 178(66) 1210-1211.

Bender, A. D., Geriatric pharmacology – a descriptive definition, **Journal of the American Geriatrics Society**, October 1966, 14(10), 1013-1015.

Bender, A. D., Gerontological basis for modifications in drug activity with age, **Journal of Pharmaceutical Sciences**, August 1965, 54(8), 1225.

Bender, A. D., Kormendy, C. G. and Powell, R., Pharmacological control of aging, **Experimental Gerontology**, July 1970, 5(2), 97-129.

Bender, A. D., Pharmacodynamic consequences of aging and their implications in the treatment of the elderly patient, **Medical Annals (District of Columbia)**, May 1967, 36(5), 267-271.

Bender, A. D., Pharmacologic aspects of aging: additional literature, **Journal of the American Geriatrics Society**, January 1967, 15(1), 68-74.

Benson, H., Decreased alcohol intake associated with practice of meditation: a retrospective investigation, **Annals of the New York Academy of Sciences**, April 1974, 233, 174-177.

Benson, Herbert, **The Relaxation Response**, New York: Avon Books, 1976.

Benson, H., Kotch, J. B. and Crassweller, K. D., Stress and hypertension: interrelations and management, **Cardiovascular Clinics**, 1978, 9(1), 113-124.

Benson, H., Greenwood, M. M. and Klemchuk, H., The relaxation response: psychophysiologic aspects and clinical applications, **International Journal of Psychiatry Medicine**, 1975, 6(1-2), 87-98.

Benson, H., Kotch, J. B. and Crassweller, K. D., The relaxation response: a bridge between psychiatry and medicine, **Medical Clinics of North America**, July 1977, 61(4), 929-938.

Benson, H., Melvea, B. P., and Graham, J. R., Physiologic correlates of meditation and their clinical effects in headache: an ongoing investigation, **Headache**, April 1973, 13(1), 23-24.

Benson, H., Rosner, B. A., Marzetta, B. R. and Klemchuk, H. P., Decreased blood pressure in borderline hypertensive subjects who practiced meditation, **Journal of Chronic Disease**, March 1974, 27(3), 163-169.

Berkal, J. and DeWaard, F., Mortality pattern and life expectancy of Seventh-Day Adventists in the Netherlands, **International Journal of Epidemiology**, Dec. 1983, 12(4), 455-459.

Bialer, I., Conceptualization of success and failure in mentally retarded and normal children, **Journal of Personality**, 1971, 39, 407-19.

Bigelow, E. A., The effects of consumer education and decision- making skill instruction on locus of control orientation and career maturity of high school seniors, Unpublished doctoral dissertation, Boston University 1981.

Blauer, Stephen, **Rejuvenation**, Santa Monica, California: Green Grown Publications, 1980.

Bonjour, J. P., Biotin in Man's nutrition and therapy – a review, **International Journal of Vitamin and Nutritional Research**, 47:107, 1977.

Borkan, G. A. and Norris, A. H., Assessment of biological age using a profile of physical parameters, **Journal of Gerontology**, 1980 March 35(2), 177-184.

Bradley, M. O., Erickson, L. C. and Kohn, K. W., Normal DNA strand rejoining and absence of DNA crosslinking in proseroid and aging human cells, **Mutation Research**, November 1976, 37(2-3), 279-292.

Bramwell, S. T., Masuda, M., Wagner, N. N. and Holmes, T. H., Psychosocial factors in athletic injuries: development and application of the social and athletic readjustment rating scale, **Journal of Human Stress**, June 1975, 1(2).

Broustet, J. P., Bellegrin, J. L., Groulier, J. I., Barbier, R. and Pir, A., General considerations on the advantages and pitfalls of exercise testing in the evaluation of cardiac failure, **European Heart Journal**, January 1983, 4(A), 107-114.

Broustet, J. P., Coue, J. C., Pir, A., Saliou, B. and Guern, P., Predictive value of symptom-limited exercise testing for life expectancy in inoperable coronary patients with disabling angina, **Cardiology** , 1981, 68(2), 114-123.

Brown, W. A. and Heningerr, G., Stress-induced growth hormone release: Psychologic and physiologic correlates, **Psychosomatic Medicine**, 1976, 38:145-147.

Bruce, R. A., Exercise, functional aerobic capacity, and aging – another viewpoint, **Medical Science of Sports Exercise**, 1984, 16(1), 8-13.

Bruder, Roy, **Discovering Natural Foods**, Santa Barbara, California: Woodbridge Press Publishing Company, 1982.

Bry, Adelaide, **How to Get Angry Without Feeling Guilty**, New York, New York: New American Library, 1976.

Bry, Adelaide, with Bair, Marjorie, **VISUALIZATION: Directing the Movies of Your Mind**, New York, New York: Barnes & Noble Books, 1978.

Burkitt, D. P., Cancer of the colon and rectum. Epidemiology and possible causative factors, **Minnesota Medicine**, September 1972, 55(9), 779-783.

Burkitt, D. P., Epidemiology of cancer of the colon and rectum, **Cancer**, July 1971, 28(1), 3-13.

Burkitt, D. P., Walker, A.R.P. and Painter, N.S., Dietary fiber and disease, **Journal of the American Medical Association**, August 1974, 229(8), 1068-1074.

Burns, George, **How to Live to be 100 – Or More: The Ultimate Diet, Sex and Exercise Book**, New York, New York: New American Library, 1983.

Burns, K. L., Social learning theory and behavioral health care, **Psychotherapy and Psychosomatics**, 1979, 32(1-4), 6-15.

Cameron, E. and Campbell, A., The orthomolecular treatment of cancer II. Clinical trial of high dose ascorbic acid supplements in advanced human cancer, **Chemical-Biological Interactions**, 1974, Vol. 9, 285-315.

Cameron, E. and Pauling, L., Ascorbic acid and the glycosaminoglycans. An orthomolecular approach to cancer and other diseases, **Oncology**, 1973, 27(2), 181-192.

Cameron, E. and Rotman, D., Ascorbic acid, cell proliferation, and cancer, **Lancet**, March 1972, 1(749), 542.

Carroll, K. K., Experimental evidence of dietary factors and hormone-dependent cancers, **Cancer Research**, November 1975, Vol. 35, 3374-3382.

Carroll, K. K., The role of dietary protein in hypercholesterolemia and atherosclerosis, **Lipids**, May 1978, 13(5), 360-365.

Cassel, Russell N., **The Psychology of Decision Making**, North Quincy, MA: The Christopher Publishing House, 1973.

Cheraskin, Emmanuel, Ringsdorf, Marshall, Jr., and Sisley, Emily L., The amazing healing properties of vitamin C, **Vegetarian Times**, September 1984, 24-26, 58.

Cherkin, A. and Eckardt, M. J., Effects of dimerhylaminoethanol upon life span and behavior of aged Japanese Quail, **Journal of Gerontology**, January 1977, Vol. 12, 38-45.

Christie, M. J. and Venables, P. H., Basal palmar skin potential and the electrocardiogram T-wave, **Psychophysiology**, November 1971, 8(6), 779-786.

Christie, M. J. and Venables, P. H., Characteristics of palmar skin potential and conductance in relaxed human subjects, **Psychophysiology**, July 1971, 8(4), 525-532.

Cohen, B. J., Dietary factors affecting rats used in aging research, **Journal of Gerontology**, November 1979, 34(6), 803-807.

Cohen, M. J., Rickles, W. H. and McArthur, D. L, Evidence for physiological response stereotypy in migraine headache, **Psycholosomatic Medicine**, June 1978, 40(4), 344-354.

Coleman, M. and Thompson, T. R., A possible role of vitamin E in the prevention or amelioration of bronchopulmonary dysplasia. **American Journal of Pediatric Hematology/Oncology**, Summer 1979, 1(2), 175-178.

Combs, G. F. Jr., Noguchi, T. and Scott, M. L., Mechanisms of action of selenium and vitamin E in protection of biological membranes, **Federation Proceedings**, October 1975, 34(11), 2090-2095.

Comfort, A., Accelerated ageing in young mothers of children with Down's syndrome, **Lancet**, September 1972, 2(776), 537.

Comfort, A., Dayan, A. D. and Wilson, J., A new line on age pigment?,**Lancet**, November 1970, 2(683), 1143.

Comfort, A., Effect of procaine on ageing, **Lancet**, May 1973, 1(183), 1193.

Comfort, A., Physiology, homeostasis and ageing,**Gerontologia**, 1968, 14(4), 224-234.

Comfort, A., Test-battery to measure ageing-rate in man, **Lancet**, December 1969, 2(635), 1411-1414.

Comfort, A., The position of aging studies, **Mechanical Ageing Development**, March 1974, 3(1), 1-31.

Comfort, A., Youthotsky, Gore I. and Pathmanathan, K., Effect of ethoxyquin on the longevity of C3H mice, **Nature**, January 1971, 229(282), 254-255.

The Complete Runner, by the editors of **Runner's World** magazine, New York, New York: Avon Books, 1974.

Conklin, Robert, **How To Get People To Do Things**, New York, New York: Ballantine Books, 1979.

Cooper, Kenneth H., **The Aerobics Program For Total Well-Being**, New York, New York: Bantam Books, 1982.

Cooper, K.H., Pollock, M.L., Martin, R.P., et al., Physical fitness levels vs selected coronary risk factors: A cross- sectional study,**Journal of the American Medical Association**, 1976, Vol. 236, 165-169.

Cott, Allan, with Agel, Jerome and Boe, Eugene, **Fasting as a Way of Life**, New York, New York: Bantam Books, 1977.

Cotzias, G. C., Miller, S. T., Nicholson, A. R. Jr, Matson, W. H. and Tang, L. C., Prolongation of the life-span in mice adapted to large amounts of L-dopa, **Proceedings of the National Academy of Science – U.S.A.**, June 1974, 71(6), 2466-2469.

Cotzias, G.C., Miller, S.T., Tang, L.C., et al., Levodopa fertility, and longevity, **Science**, April 1977, Vol. 196, 549-550.

Coulehan, J. L., et al., Vitamin C and acute illness in Navajo school children, **New England Journal of Medicine**, 1976, 295:973.

Cowan, G. J., The effects of teaching goal-setting procedures on the career maturity and classroom performance of business college women differing in locus of control, Unpublished doctoral dissertation, Boston University, 1979.

Crouse, J. R., Grundy, S. M. and Ahrens, E. H. Jr., Cholesterol distribution in the bulk tissues of man: variation with age, **Journal of Clinical Investigations**, May 1972, 51(5), 1292-1296.

Curry, J. A., The effects of life planning instruction and career counseling on locus of control orientation and career maturity scores of university compensatory education students, Unpublished doctoral dissertation, Boston University, 1980.

Davies, J. E., Ellery, P. M., Heyworth, P. G. and Hughes, R. E., The influence of ingested flouride on the ascorbic acid concentration in guinea-pig tissues, **Experientia**, April 1978, 34(4), 429.

Davies, J. E. W., Ellery, P. M. and Hughes, R. E., Dietary ascorbic acid and life span of guinea pigs, **Experimental Gerontology**, 1977, 12(5-6), 215-216.

DeCosse, J.J., Condon, R.E. and Adams, M.B., Surgical and medical measures in prevention of large bowel cancer, **Cancer**, May, 1977, Vol. 40, 2549-2552.

Denckla, D. W., A time to die, **Life Sciences**, January 1975, 16(1), 31-44.

DeVries, H. A. and Adams, G. M., Comparison of exercise responses in old and young men: I. The cardiac effort-total body effort relationship, **Journal of Gerontology**, July 1972, 27(3), 344-348.

DeVries, H. A. and Adams, G. M., Comparison of exercise responses in old and young men: II. Ventilatory mechanics, **Journal of Gerontology**, July 1972, 27(3), 349-352.

Doll, R. and Peto, R., Mortality among doctors in different occupations, **British Medical Journal**, June 1977, 1(6074), 1433-1436.

Doll, R. and Peto, R., Mortality in relation to smoking: 20 years' observations on male British doctors, **British Medical Journal**, December 25, 1976, Vol. 2, 1525-1536.

Dong, M. H. et al., Thiamin, riboflavin and vitamin B6 contents of selected foods as served, **Journal of the American Dietetic Association**, 1980, 76:156.

Dormandy, T. L., Free-radical oxidation and antioxidants, **Lancet**, March 1978, 1(8065), 647-650.

Downs, Robert W., with VanBaak, Alice, ZINC! Proven natural remedies help protect us in extremely important ways. One of these is the mineral zinc, **Bestways**, June 1984, 20,23.

Drachman, D. A. and Leavitt, J., Human memory and the cholinergic system. A relationship to aging?, **Archives of Neurology**, 1974, 30(2), 113-121.

Drachman, D. A., Memory and cognitive function in man: does the cholinergic system have a specific role?, **Neurology**, August 1977 27(8), 783-790.

Drake, J. R. and Fitch, C. O., Status of Vitamin E as an erythropoietic factor, **American Journal of Clinical Nutrition**, 1980, 33:2386.

Dyer, Wayne W., **Pulling Your Own Strings**, New York, New York: Avon Books, 1977.

Dyer, Wayne W., **Your Erroneous Zones**, New York, New York: Avon Books, 1976.

Ehrenkranz, R. A. et al., Amelioration of bronchopulmonary dysplasia after Vitamin E administration, **New England Journal of Medicine**, 1978, 299:564.

Ehret, Arnold, **Mucusless-Diet Healing System**, Cody, Wyoming: Ehret Literature Publishing Co., 1953.

Ellestad-Sayed, J. J., Nelson, R. A., Adson, M. A., Palmer, W. M. and Soule, E. H., Pantothenic acid, coenzyme A, and human chronic ulcerative and granulomatous colitis, **American Journal of Clinical Nutrition**, December 1976, 29(12), 1333- 1338.

Elliot, R. S., Stress and cardiovascular disease, **European Journal of Cardiology**, March 1977, 5(2), 97-104.

Enesco, H. E. and Samborsky, J., Liver: polyploidy: influence of age and of dietary restriction, **Experimental Gerontology**, 1983, 18(1), 79-87.

Engleman, Laura, Megavitamin therapies yield promising results, **Vegetarian Times**, Issue #54, 28-31.

Epstein, L., Miller, G.J., Stitt, F.W., et al., Vigorous exercise in leisure time, coronary risk-factors, and resting electrocardiogram in middle-aged male civil servants,**British Heart Journal**, 1976, Vol. 38, 403-409.

Eyton, Audrey, **The F-Plan Diet**, New York, New York: Crown Publishers, Inc., 1982.

Fensterheim, Herbert and Baer, Jean, **Don't Say Yes When You Want To Say No**, New York, New York: Dell Publishing Co., Inc., 1975.

Fernstrom, J. D. and Wurtman, R. J., Nutrition and the brain, **Scientific American**, February 1974, 230(2), 84-91.

Finch, C. E., Catecholamine metabolism in the brains of ageing male mice, **Brain Research**, March 1973, 52, 261-176.

Fiske, Marjorie, **Middle Age the prime of life?**, New York, New York: Harper & Row, 1979.

Foley, Denise, Vitamin E healing update, **Prevention**, May 1984, 20-23.

Frankel, B. L., Patel, D. J., Horwitz, D., Friedewald, W. T. and Gaarder, K. R., Treatment of hypertension with biofeedback and relaxation techniques, **Psychosomatic Medicine**, June 1978, 40(4), 276-293.

Freis, E.D., Salt, volume and the prevention of hypertension, **Circulation**, April 1976, Vol.53, 589-595.

Frumkin, K.,Nathan, R. J., Prout, M. F. and Cohen, M. C., Nonpharmacologic control of essential hypertension in man: A critcal review of the experimental literature. **Psychosomatic Medicine**, June 1978, 40(4), 294-320.

Fryer, F. W., **Evaluation of Level of Aspiration As A Training Procedure**, Inglewood Cliffs, New Jersey: Prentice-Hall, 1964.

Funderburk, James, **Science Studies Yoga**, Honesdale, Pennsylvania: The Himalayan International Institute of Yoga Science & Philosophy of USA, 1977.

Furukawa, T., Inoue, M., Kajiya, F., Inada, H. and Takasugi, S., Assessment of biological age by multiple regression analysis, **Journal of Gerontology**, July 1975, 30(4), 422-434.

Gardner, D. C., Beatty, G. J., & Bigelow, E. A., Locus of control and career maturity: A pilot evaluation of a life-planning and career development program for high school students, **Adolescence**, XVI(63), Fall, 1981.

Gardner, D. C. & Beatty, G. J., Locus of control change techniques: Important variables in work training, **Education**, Spring 1980, 100(3):237-242.

Gardner, D. C. & Beatty G. J., Personality characteristics and learning styles of disadvantaged youth: Important considerations in teaching job related language and developing work attitudes, Paper presented at the Leadership Training Institute on CETA/Vocational Education and Vocational Rehabilitation Linkages, Hartford, Connecticut: Sheraton-Hartford Hotel, May 4-6, 1980.

Gardner, D. C., Career maturity and locus of control: Important factors in career training, **College Student Journal, Fall 1981, 15(3):239-246.**

Gardner, D. C. & Gardner, P. L., Goal-setting and learning in the high school resource room, **Adolescence**, 1974, 18(51): 489-493.

Gardner, D.C., Goal setting, locus of control, and work performance of mentally retarded adults, Unpublished doctoral dissertation, Boston University, 1974.

Gardner D. C., Warren, S. A. and Gardner, P. L., Locus of control and law knowledge: a comparison of normal, retarded and learning disabled adolescents, **Adolescence**, 1977, 12(45), 103-109.

Gardner, D. C. & Warren, S. A., **Careers and Disabilities: A Career Education Approach**, Stamford, Connecticut: Greylock Publishers, 1978.

Garfield, Charles A. and Bennett, Hal Zina, Soviet Shamans in Milan, **East West Journal**, August 1984, 41-43.

Gelb, Micahel, **Body Learning**, New York, New York: Delilah Books, 1981.

Gentleman, J.F. and Forbes, W. F., Cancer mortality for males and females and its relation to cigarette smoking, **Journal of Gerontology**, May 1974, 29(5), 518-533.

Georgieff, K. K., Free radical inhibitory effect of some anticancer compounds, **Science**, August 1971, 173(996), 537-539.

Gerbase, DeLima, M., Liu, R. K., Cheney, K. E., Mickey, R. and Walford, R. L., Immune function and survival in a long-lived mouse strain subjected to undernutrition, **Gerontology**, 1975, 21(4), 184-202.

Gergan, Kenneth J., and Marlowe, David (editors), **Personality and Social Behavior**, Reading, Masschusetts: Addison-Wesley Publishing Company, 1970.

Gessa, G. L. and Tagliamonte, A., Role of brain monoamines in male sexual behavior, **Life Sciences**, 1974, 14(3), 425-436.

Gilmore, John V., **The Productive Personality**, San Francisco, California: Albion Publishing Company, 1974.

Ginter, E., Cholesterol: Vitamin C controls its transformation to bile acids, **Science**, February 1973, 179(74), 702-704.

Goldman, J. and Plotnik, M., Aging: the criterion problem in diagnosis of brain dysfunction, **Journal of Gerontology**, January 1967, 23(1), 34.

Goodman, Hal, Eat, drink and be wary, **Psychology Today**, August 1984, 17.

Goodrick, C. L. et al., Effects of intermittent feeding upon growth, activity, and lifespan in rats allowed voluntary exercise, **Experimental Aging Research**, 1983, 9(3), 203-209.

Goodrick, C.L., The effects of exercise on longevity and behavior of hybrid mice which differ in coat color, **Journal of Gerontology**, February 1974, 29(2), 129-133.

Grande, F. and Prisse, W. F., Serum lipid changes produced in dose by substituting coconut oil for either sucrose or protein in the diet, **Journal of Nutrition**, May 1974, 104(5), 613-618.

Green, L. W., Modifying and developing health behavior, **Annual Review of Public Health**, 1984 5, 215-236.

Greenwood, M. M. and Benson, H., The efficacy of progressive relaxation in systematic desensitization and a proposal for an alternative competitive response – the relaxation response, **Behavioral Research Theory**, 1977, 15(4), 337-343.

Gregory, Dick, **Dick Gregory's Natural Diet for Folks Who Eat: Cookin' with Mother Nature**, New York, New York: Harper & Row Publishers, Inc., 1973.

Gross, Joy, The tast way to rejuvenate body & spirit, **Vegetarian Times**, June 1984, 32, 34-36.

Haeger, K., Letter: Vitamin E in intermittent claudication, **Lancet**, June 1974, 1(870), 1352.

Haeger, K., Long-time treatment of intermittent claudication with vitamin E, **American Journal of Clinical Nutrition**, October 1974, 27(10), 1179-1181.

Haeger, K., Vitamin E in peripheral blood vessel insufficiency, **Tidsskrift For Den Norske Laegeforening**, November 1970, 90(22), 2112-2114.

Haeger, K., Walking distance and arterial flow during long term treatment of intermittent claudication with d-a-tocopherol, **Vascularity**, 1973, 2(3), 28-287.

Halsted, C. H., The intestinal absorption of folates, **American Journal of Clinical Nutrition**, 1976, 32:846.

Hamermesh, D. S. and Hamermesh, F. W., Does perception of life expectancy reflect health knowledge?, **American Journal of Public Health**, August 1983, 73(8), 911-914.

Hareer, A. F., Coronary heart disease – an epidemic related to diet?, **American Journal of Clinical Nutrition**, April 1983, 37(4), 669-681.

Harman, D. and Eddy, D. L., Free radical theory of aging: Effect of adding antioxidants to maternal mouse diets on the lifespan of the offspring, **Age**, 1978, 1:162.

Harman, D. and Piette, L. H., Free radical theory of aging: free radical reactions in serum, **Journal of Gerontology**, October 1966, 21(4), 560-565.

Harman, D., Curtis, H. J. and Tilley, J., Chromosomal aberrations in liver cells of mice fed free radical reaction inhibitors, **Journal of Gerontology**, January 1970, 25(1), 17-19.

Harman, D., Eddy, D. E. and Noffsinger, J., Free radical theory of aging: inhibition of amyloidosis in mice by antioxidants; possible mechanism, **Journal of the American Geriatrics Society**, May 1976, 24(5), 203-210.

Harman, D., Heidrick, M. L. and Eddy. D. E., Free radical theory of aging: Effect of free-radical-reaction inhibitors on the immune response, **Journal of the American Geriatrics Society**, September 1977, 25(9), 400-407.

Harman, D, Henricks, S., Eddy, D. E. and Seibold, J., Free radical theory of aging: Effect of dietary fat on central nervous system function, **Journal of the American Geriatrics Society**, July 1976, 24(7), 301-307.

Harman, D., Free radical theory of aging: effect of free radical reaction inhibitors on the mortality rate of male LAF mice, **Journal of Gerontology**, October 1968, 23(4), 476-482.

Harman, D., Free radical theory of aging: Origin of life, evolution, and aging, **Age**, 3:100 (1980).

Harman, D., Nutritional implications of the free-radical theory of aging, **Journal of American College Nutrition**, 1982, 1(1), 27-34.

Harman, D., Prolongation of life: role of free radical reactions in aging, **Journal of the American Geriatrics Society**, August 1969, 17(8), 721-735.

Harman, D., The aging process, **Proceedings of the National Academy of Science--U.S.A.**, November 1981, 78(11), 7124-7128.

Hart, R. W. and Setlow, R. B., Correlation between DNA excision-repair and lifespan in a number of mammalian species, **Proceedings of the National Academy of Science**, June 1974, 71(6): 2169-2173.

Hausman, Patricia, Fighting cancer with nutrition, **Runner's World**, June 1984, 59-62, 78.

Haussler, M. R. and McCain, T. A., Basic and clinical concepts related to vitamin D metabolism and action (first of two parts), **New England Journal of Medicine**, November 1977, 297(18), 974-983.

Haussler, M. R. and McCain, T. A., Basic and clinical concepts related to vitamin D metabolism and action (second of two parts), **New England Journal of Medicine**, November 1977, 297(19), 1041-1050.

Hayflick, L., Future directions in ageing research, **Proceedings of the Society of Experimental Biological Medicine**, Nov. 1980, 165(2), 106-214.

Hayflick, L., Human cells and aging, **Science American**, March 1968, 218(3), 32-37.

Heart disease, often a family affair, **Vegetarian Times**, March 1984, 8.

Henderson, Joe, **Jog, Run, Race**, Mountain View, California: World Publications, 1977.

Henker, R. O. III, Neurologic disease in elderly psychoneurotics, **Southern Medical Journal**, October 1968, 61(10), 1042-1044.

Herbert, V., Jacob, E., Wong, K. T., Scott, J. and Pfeffer, R. D., Low serum Vitamin B12 levels in patients receiving ascorbic acid in megadoses: Studies concerning the effect of ascorbate on radioisotope Vitamin B12 Assay, **American Journal of Clinical Nutrition**, February 1978, 31(2), 253-258.

Hinton, J., Whom do dying patients tell?, **Boston Medical Journal**, Nov. 1980, 281(6251) 1328-1330.

Hittleman, Richard L., **Be Young With Yoga**, New York, New York: Paperback Library, Inc., 1962.

Hochberg, Arthur, How to reduce stress with simple dietary changes, **Vegetarian Times**, September 1984, 28, 49.

Hochschild, R., Effect of dimethylaminoethyl p-chlorophenoxyacetate on the life span of male Swiss Webster Albino mice, **Experimental Gerontology**, August 1973, 8(4), 177-183.

334

Hochschild, R., Effects of various drugs on longevity in female C57BL/6J mice, **Gerontology**, 1973, 19(5), 271-280.

Hogenkamp, H. P. C., The interactions between vitamins B12 and vitamin C, **American Journal of Clinical Nutrition**, 33:1, 1980.

Holmes, T. H. and Rahe, R. H., (1976), The social readjustment rating scale, **Journal of Psychosomatic Research**, 1967, 11(2), 213-218.

Hopkins, G. J. and West, C. E., Possible roles of dietary fats in carcinogenesis, **Life Sciences**, October 1976, 19(8), 1103-1116.

Hopkins, G. J. and West, C. E., Effect of dietary polyunsaturated fat on the growth of the transplantable adnocarcinoma in C3HAvyfB mice, **Journal of the National Cancer Institute**, March 1977, 58(3), 753-756.

Hopkins, G. J., Hard, G. C. and West, C. E., Carcinogenesis induced by 7,12-dimethylbenz(a)anthracene in c3H-A vyfB mice: influence of different dietary fats, **Journal of the National Cancer Institute**, April 1978, 60(4), 849-853.

House, James S., **Work Stress and Social Support**, Reading, Massachusetts: Addison-Wesley Publishing Company, 1981.

Howard, R. B. and Herbold, N. H., **Nutrition In Clinical Care**, New York, New York: McGraw-Hill Book Company, 1982.

Hruza, Z. and Zbuzkova, V., Decrease of excretion of cholesterol during aging, **Experimental Gerontology**, February 1973, 8(1), 29-37.

Hruza, Z., Effect of endocrine factors on cholesterol turnover in young and old rats, **Experimental Gerontology**, June 1971, 6(3), 199-204.

Hruza, Z., Increase of cholesterol turnover of old rats connected by parabiosis with young rats, **Experimental Gerontology**, June 1971, 6(3), 199-204.

Jacobs. E. A., Alvis, H. J., and Small, S. M., Hyperoxygenation: A central nervous system activator?, **Journal of Geriatric Psychiatry**, 1972, 5(2), 107-136.

Janney, J. G., Masuda, M. and Holmes, T. H., Impact of a natural catastrophe on life events, **Journal of Human Stress**, June 1977, 3(2), 22-34.

Johnson, Kirk, Can foods improve your memory?, **East West Journal**, August 1984, 56-60.

Johnson, Robert A., **SHE, Understanding Feminine Psychology**, New York, New York: Harper & Row, 1976.

Johnson, Robert A., **HE, Understanding Masculine Psychology**, New York, New York: Harper & Row, 1974.

Jolma, V. H. and Hruza, Z., Differences in properties of newly formed collagen during aging and parabiosis, **Journal of Gerontology**, April 1972, 27(2), 178-182.

Jones, F. P., Method of changing stereotyped response patterns by the inhibition of certain postural sets, **Psychological Review**, 1965, 70(3), 196-214.

Jose, D. G., Stutman, O., Good, R. A., Long-term effects on immune function of early nutritional deprivation, **Nature**, January 1973, 241(384), 57-58.

Jussek, E. G. and Roscher, A. A., Critical review of contemporary cellular therapy (Celltherapy), **Journal of Gerontology**, April 1970, 25(2), 119-125.

Kabuto, Michnori, Biological aging in down's syndrome, **Journal of Mental Health**, March 1979, 26, 57-68.

Katz, Jane, with Bruning, Nancy P., **Swimming For Total Fitness**, Garden City, New York: Dolphin Books/Doubleday & Company, Inc., 1981.

Kausler, D. H., Aspiration level as a determinant of performance, **Journal of Personality**, 1959, 27, 356-361.

Kay, R. M. and Truswell, A. S., Effect of citrus pectin on blood lipids and fecal steroid excretion in man, **American Journal of Clinical Nutrition**, February 1977, 30(2), 171-175.

Kent, D. C. and Cenci, L., Smoking and the workplace: tobacco smoke health hazards to the involuntary smoker, **Journal of Medicine**, June 1982, 24(6), 469-472.

Kent, S., Body weight and life expectancy, **Geriatrics**, Feb. 1982, 37(2), 149-157.

Kent, S., Do free radicals and dietary antioxidants wage intracellular war?, **Geriatrics**, January 1977, 32(1), 127-136.

Kilhman, Christopher, **The Complete Shoppers' Guide To Natural Foods**, Brookline, Massachusetts: The Autumn Press, 1980.

Kimball, C. P., A predictive study of adjustment to cardiac surgery, **Journal of Thoracic and Cardiovascular Surgery**, December 1969, 58(6), 891-896.

Kirban, Salem, **How Juices Restore Health NATURALLY**, Huntingdon Valley, Pennsylvania: Salem Kirban, Inc., 1980.

Kirschner, H. E., **Live Food Juices**, Monrovia, California: H. E. Kirschner Publications, 1957.

Klevay, L. M., Coronary heart disease: The zinc/copper hypothesis. **American Journal of Clinical Nutrition**, July 1975, 28(7), 764-774.

Kliebhan, J. M., Effects of goal-setting and modeling on job performance of retarded adolescents, **American Journal of Mental Deficiency**, 1967, 72(2), 220-226.

Kobasa, S. C., Stressful life events, personality and health: An inquiry into hardiness, **Journal of Personality and Social Psychology**, January 1979, 37(1), 1-11.

Kohn, R. R., Effect of antioxidants on life-span of C57BL mice, **Journal of Gerontology**, July 1971, 26(3), 378-380.

Koloszey, Jody, Life gets better as we get older, **Prevention**, August 1982, 30-32.

Koloszey, Jody, Nutrients to help uncramp your style, **Prevention**, November 1982, 143, 145-148.

Konishi, F. and Harrison, S.L., Vitamin D for adults, **Journal of Nutrition Education**, 11:120, 1980.

Konoplya, E. F., Dubina, T. L., Zelezinskaya, G. A., Dyundikova, V. A., Pokrovskaya, R. V., Gulko, V. V., Mazhul, L. M. and Gatsko, G. G., Vitamins and periodic fasting as possible factors of experimental prolongation of life span, **Fiziologiya i Biokhimiya Kul'turnykh Rastenii**, 1984, 30(1), 16-24.

Kormendy, C. G. and Bender, A. D., Chemical interference with aging, **Gerontology**, 17(1), 52-64.

Kormendy, C. G. and Bender, A. D., Experimental modification of the chemistry and biology of the aging process, **Journal of Pharmaceutical Sciences**, February 1971, 60(2), 167-180.

Kothari, L. K., Bordia, A. and Gupta, O. P., Studies on a Yogi during an eight-day confinement in a sealed underground pit, **Indian Journal of Medical Research**, November 1973, 61(11), 1645-1650.

Kushi, Michio and the East West Foundation, **The Macrobiotic Approach to Cancer**, Wayne, New Jersey: Avery Publishing Group, Inc., 1982.

Kushi, Michio, **The Book of Macrobiotics**, Tokyo, Japan: Japan Publications, 1977.

Landis, Pat Murphy, Bringing Yoga to the elderly, **Yoga Journal**, September/October, 16-18.

Lave, L.B. and Seskin, E. P., Air pollution, climate and home heating: their effects on U.S. mortality rates?, **American Journal of Public Health**, July 1972, 62(7), 909-916.

Lee, William H., **The Book of Raw Fruit and Vegetable Juices and Drinks**, New Canaan, Connecticut: Keats Publishing.

Leepson, Marc, **Alive & Well Stress Book**, New York, New York: Bantam Books, 1984.

Lefcourt, Herbert M., **Locus Of Control Current Trends in Theory and Research**, Hillsdale, New Jersey: Lawrence Erlbaum Associates, Publishers, 1976.

Lefcourt, H. M., Internal vs. external control of reinforcement: A review, **Psychological Bulletin**, 1966, 66(4), 206-220.

Legros, J. J., Gilot, P., Seron, X., Claeggens, J., Adam, A., Moeglen, J. M., Audibert, A. and Berchier, P., Influence of vasopressin on memory and learning, **Lancet**, January 1978, 1(8054), 41-42.

Leibel, R. L., Behavioral and biochemical correlates of iron deficiency, **Journal of the American Diet Association**, October 1977, 71(4), 398-404.

Levi, Lennart, **Preventing Work Stress**, Reading, Massachusetts: Addison-Wesley Publishing Company, 1981.

Lewin, K., Dembo, T., Festinger, L., Sears, P., Level of aspiration in: J. McV. Hunt (ed.), **Personality and the Behavior Disorders**, New York: Ronald Press, 1944, 333-378.

Lippman, R. D., The prolongation of life: a comparison of antioxidants and geroprotectors versus superoxide in human mitochondria, **Journal of Gerontology**, September 1981, 36(5), 550-557.

Lipson, Goldie, **Rejuvenation Through Yoga**, New York, New York: Pyramid Books, 1963.

Little, J. B., Relationship between DNA repair capacity and cellular aging, **Gerontology**, 1976, 22(1-2), 28-55.

Little, S. W. and Cohen, L.D., Goal setting behavior of asthmatic children, and of their mothers for them, **Journal of Personality**, 1951, 19, 376-389.

Liu, R.K., and Walford R.L., Mid-life temperature-transfer effects on life span of annual fish, **Journal of Gerontology**, March 1975, 30(2), 129-131.

Liu R. K. and Walford, R. L., Observations on the lifespans of several species of annual fishes and of the world's smallest fishes, **Experimental Gerontology**, September 1970, 5(3), 241-246.

Liu, R.K. and Walford, R.L., The effect of lowered body temperature on lifespan and immune and nonimmune processes, **Gerontology**, 1972, 18(5-6), 363-388.

Liu, R. K., Leung, B. E. and Walford, R. L., Effect of temperature-transfer on growth of laboratory populations of a South American annual fish Cynolebias bellottii, **Growth**, September 1975, 39(3), 337-343.

Lockette, R. E., The effect of level of aspiration upon learning skills, Unpublished doctoral dissertation, University of Illinois, 1956.

Lowe, Carl and Nechas, James, et al., **Whole body Healing**, Emmaus, Pennsylvania: Rodale Press, 1983.

Lust, John B., **The Herb Book**, New York, New York: Bantam Books, 1974.

Lynch, J. J., Paskewitz, D. A., Gimbel, K. S. and Thomas, S. A., Psychological aspects of cardiac arrhythmia, **American Heart Journal**, May 1977, 93(5), 645-657.

Lynch, J. J., Thomas, S. A., Paskewitz, D. A., Katcher, A. H. and Weir, L. O., Human contact and cardiac arrhythmia in a coronary care unit, **Psychosomatic Medicine**, May/June 1977, 39(3), 188-192.

Madorsky, J. G. Radford, L. M. and Newmann, E. M., Psychosocial aspects of death and dying in Duchenne muscular dystrophy. **Archives of Physical Medicine and Rehabilitation**, February, 1984, 65(2), 79-82.

Mager, Robert F. and Pipe, Peter, **Analyzing Performance Problems**, Belmont, California: Fearon Pitman Publishers, Inc., 1970.

Makinodan, T., Control of immunologic abnormalities associated with ageing, **Mechanisms of Ageing and Development**, January 1979, 9(1-2), 7-17.

Maleskey, Gale, On the mend with vitamins and minerals, **Prevention**, June 1984, 75-80.

Mallia, A. K, Smith, J. E. and Goodman, D. W., Metabolism of retinol-binding protein and vitamin A during hypervitaminosis A in the rat, **Journal of Lipid Research**, May 1975, 16(3), 180-188.

Mann, G. V., A factor in yogurt which lowers cholesteremia in man, **Atherosclerosis**, March 1977, 26(3), 335-340.

Marano, Hara Estroff, Blood, sweat, tears....& laughter, **American Health**, November/December 1983, 50-55.

Marquardt, H., Rufino, F., and Weisburger, J.H., Mutagenic activity of nitrite treated foods: Human stomach cancer may be related to dietary factors, **Science**, May 1977, 196(4293), 1000-1001.

Masuda, M. and Holmes, T. H., Life events: perceptions and frequencies, **Psychosomatic Medicine**, May 1978, 40(3), 236- 261.

Mazer, Eileen, 12 Ways to lower your blood pressure naturally, **Prevention**, July 1982, 129-134.

Mazer, Eileen, Nutritional fuel for a lead-free life, **Prevention**, October 1982, 139-142, 144, 146.

Mazess, R. B. and Forman, S. H., Longevity and age exaggeration in Vilcabamba, Ecuador, **Journal of Gerontology**, January 1979, 34(1), 94-98.

McDougall, John and McDougall, Mary, The latest thinking on protein, **Vegetarian Times**, August 1984, 24-26, 28.

McLean, Alan A., **Work Stress**, Reading, Massachusetts: Addison-Wesley Publishing Company, 1979.

Medovar, B., Effects of a diet with various protein contents on the life span of rats, **Voprosy Virusologii**, Nov-Dec 1983, (6) 56-8.

Meichenbaum, Donald, **Cognitive-Behavior Modification**, New York, New York: Plenum Press, 1977.

Meichenbaum, D., Ways of modifying what clients say to themselves, **Ontario Psychologist**, 1972, 4(3), 144-151.

Meites, J., Steger, R. W. and Hauang, H. H., Relation of neuroendocrine system to the reproductive decline in aging rats and human subjects, **Federation Proceedings**, December 1980, 39(14), 3168-3172.

Merari, A. and Ginton, A., Characteristics of exaggerated sexual behavior induced by electrical stimulation of the medial preoptic area in male rats, **Brain Research**, March 1975, 86(1), 97-108.

Mertens, D.J., Shepard, R.J., and Kavanagh, T., Long-term exercise therapy for chronic obstructive lung disease, **Respiration**, 1978, 35(2), 96-107.

Miller, Jean Baker, **Toward a New Psychology of Women**, Boston, Massachusetts: Beacon Press, 1976.

Miller, N. E. and Dworkin, B. R., Effects of learning on visceral functions – biofeedback, **New England Journal of Medicine**, 296(22), 1274-1278.

Monjan, A. A. and Collector, M. I., Stress-induced modulation of the immune response, **Science**, April 1977, 197(4287), 307-308.

Monsen, E., Hallberg, L., Layrisse, M., Hegsted, D., Cook, J., Mertz, W. and Finch, C., Estimation of available dietary iron, **American Journal of Clinical Nutrition**, January 1978, 31(1), 134-141.

Monte, Tom, Heart disease a tale of two therapies, **East West Journal**, June 1984, 39-42, 44.

Moon, R. C., Thompson, H. J., Becci, P. J., Grubbs, C. J., Gander, R. J., Newton, D. L., Smith, J. M., Phillips, S. L., Henderson, W. R., Mullen, L. T., Brown, C. C. and Sporn, M. B., (4-Hydroxyphenyl)retinamide, a new retinoid for prevention of breast cancer in the rat, **Cancer Research**, April 1979, 39(4), 1339-1346.

Moore, C.J. and Schwartz, A. G., Inverse correlation between species life span and capacity to activate 7, 12-dimethylbenz(a)anthracene to a DNA-binding form (proceedings), **Advanced Experimental Medical Biology**, 1978, 97, 271.

Morris, J.N., Chave, S. P., Adam, C., Sirey, C., Epstein, L. and Sheehan, D. J., Vigorous exercise in leisure-time and the incidence of coronary heart-disease, **Lancet**, February 1973, 1(799), 333-339.

Morse, D. R., Martin, J. S., Furst, M. L. and Dubin, L. L., A physiological and subjective evaluation of meditation, hypnosis and relaxation, **Psychosomatic Medicine**, 1977, 39(5), 304-324.

Morse, D. R., Martin, J. S. Furst, M. L. and Dubin, L. L., A physiological and subjective evaluation of neutral and emotionally-charged words for meditation, Part I, **Journal of the American Society of Psychosomatic Dental Medicine**, 1979, 26(1) 31-38.

Morse, D. R., Martin, J. S., Furst, M. L. and Dubin, L. L., A physiological and subjective evaluation of neutral and emotionally-charged words for meditation, Part II, **Journal of the American Society of Psychosomatic Dental Medicine**, 1979, 26(2), 56-62.

Morse, D. R., Martin, J. S., Furst, M. L. and Dubin, L. L., A physiological and subjective evaluation of neutral and emotionally-charged words for meditation, Part III, **Journal of the American Society of Psychosomatic Dental Medicine**, 1979, 26(3), 106-112.

Moss, Leonard, **Management Stress**, Reading, Massachusetts: Addison-Wesley Publishing Company, 1981.

Muller, Rusty, The road back from cancer, **Vegetarian Times**, August 1983, 50-52.

Myers, R. D. and Yaksh, T.L., Thermoregulation around a new set-point established in the monkey by altering the ratio of sodium to calcium ions within the hypothalamus, **Journal of Physiology** (London), 1971, 218(3), 609-633.

Nandy, K., Further studies on the effects of centrophenoxine on the lipofuscin pigment in the neurons of senile guinea pigs, **Journal of Gerontology**, January 1968, 23(1), 82-92.

The new anti-cancer diet, **Vegetarian Times**, April 1984, 9.

News Digest, More accolades for fruit & vegetable rich diets, **Vegetarian Times**, July 1984, 12.

Nicholson, W. J., Cancer following occupational exposure to asbestos and vinyl chloride, **Cancer**, April 1977, 39(4 Suppl), 1792-1801.

Nierenberg, Gerard I. and Calereo, Henry H., **How to Read a Person Like a Book**, New York, New York: Pocket Books, 1971.

Nurenberger, Phil, **Freedom From Stress**, Honesdale, Pennsylvania: Himalayan International Institute of Yoga, Science and Philosophy, 1981.

Odens, M., Prolongation of the life span in rats, **Journal of the American Geriatrics Society**, October 1973, 21(10), 450-451.

Ogilvie, Bruce C. and Howe, Maynard A., Beating slumps at their game, **Psychology Today**, July 1984, 28, 30-32.

Ooka, H., Fujita, S., Yoshomoto, F., Pituitary-thyroid activity and longevity in neonatally thyroxine-treated rats, **Mechanisms of Ageing and Development**, 1983 June 22(2), 113-120.

Ornish, Dean, **Stress, Diet and Your Heart**, New York, New York: Holt, Rinehart and Winston, 1982.

Oski, F. A., Metabolism and physiologic roles of vitamin E, **Hospital Practice**, October 1977, 12(10), 79-85.

Paffenbarger, R. S. and Hale, W. E., Work activity and coronary heart mortality, **New England Journal of Medicine**, March 1975, 292(11), 545-550.

Paffenbarger, R. S. and Hyde, R. T., Exercise in the prevention of coronary heart disease, **Preview of Medicine**, January 1984, 13(1), 3-22.

Paffenbarger, R. S. Jr., Hale, W. E., Brand, R. J. and Hyde, R. T., Work energy level, personal characteristics, and fatal heart attack: a birth-cohort effect, **American Journal of Epidemiology**, March 1977, 105(3), 200-213.

Paffenbarger, R. S., Jr., Wing, A.L. and Hyde, R. T., Physical activity as an index of heart attack risk in college alumni, **American Journal of Epidemiology**, September 1978, 108(3), 161-175.

Paffenbarger, R. S. Jr., Wing, A. L., Hyde, R. T. and Jung, D. L., Physical activity and incidence of hypertension in college alumni, **American Journal of Epidemiology**, March 1983, 117(3), 245-257.

Paffenholz, V., Correlation between DNA repair of embryonic fibroblasts and different life span of 3 inbred mouse strains, **Mechanisms of Ageing and Development**, February 1978, 7(2), 131-150.

Page, L. and Friend, B., The changing USA diet, **Bioscience**, 1978, 28(3), 192-197.

Patel, Chandra, Twelve-Month follow-up of yoga and biofeedback in the management of hypertension, **Lancet**, 62(1975), ii.

Patel, C. H., Twelve-month follow-up of yoga and biofeedback in the management of hypertension, **Lancet**, 62(1975), ii.

Patel, C. H., Biofeedback-aided relaxation and meditation in the management of hypertension, **Biofeedback Self Regulation**, March 1977, 2(1), 1-41.

Pawson, I. G. and Janes, G., Biocultural risks in longevity: Samoans in California, **Social Science and Medicine**, 1982, 16(2), 183-190.

Paykel, E. S., Prusoff, B. A. and Uhlenhuth, E. H., Scaling of life events, **Archives of General Psychiatry**, October 1971, 25(4), 340-370.

Pechter, Kerry, A nutritional formula for healthy gums, **Prevention**, April 1983, 119-120, 124-126, 128.

Pechter, Kerry, How to stop diabetic complications with good nutrition, **Prevention**, June 1984, 126, 128, 145-147, 153-154.

Pechter, Kerry, Nutrition: A better way to fight alcoholism, **Prevention**, August 1983, 97-98, 100-102, 104.

Pechter, Kerry, Protect yourself from pollution with Vitamin C, **Prevention**, November 1983, 79-83.

Pechter, Kerry, Put senility in reverse with good nutrition, **Prevention**, January 1984, 77-80.

Pechter, Kerry, The psychology of successful weight loss, **Prevention**, April 1984, 35-36, 89-90, 92.

Peck, G. L., Olsen, T. G., Yoder, F. W., Strauss, J. S., Downing, D. T., Pandya, M., Butkus, D. and Arnaud-Battandier, J., Prolonged remission of cystic and conglobate acne with 13-cis-retinoic acid, **New England Journal of Medicine**, February 1979, 300(7), 329-333.

Phares, Jerry E.,**Locus of Control in Personality**, Morristown, New Jersey: General Learning Press, 1976.

Pitts, F. N. Jr., The biochemistry of anxiety, **Science American**, 220(2), 69-75.

Pollitt, E. and Leibel, R. L., Iron deficiency and behavior, **Journal of Pediatrics**, March 1976, 88(3), 372-381.

Porta, F. A., Jown, N. S. and Nitta, R. T., Effects of the type of dietary fat at two levels of vitamin E in Wistar male rats during development and aging, I. Life span, serum biochemical parameters and pathological change, **Mechanisms of Ageing and Development**, May 1980, 13(1), 1-39.

Powell, Richard, One runner's journey to better health, **Vegetarian Times**, August 1984, 20-22.

Powell, Richard, The Life of the meatless runner, **Runner's World**, May 1984, 63-65, 128.

Pritikin, N., and McGrady, P.M. Jr., **The Pritikin Program for Diet and Exercise**. New York: Grosset & Dunlap, 1979.

Pritikin, Nathan, **The Pritikin Permanent Weight-Loss Manual**, New York, New York: Bantam Books, 1981.

Rachmann, S., Marks, I. M. and Hodgson, R., The Treatment of obsessive-compulsive neurotics by modeling and flooding in vivo. **Behavior Research and Therapy**, November 1973, 11(4), 463-471.

Raven, P. B., Gettman, L. R., Pollock, M. L. and Cooper, K. H., A physiological evaluation of professional soccer players, **Journal of Sports Medicine**, December 1976, 10(4), 209-216.

Rawls, Eugene S., **A Handbook of Yoga**, New York, New York: Pyramid Books, 1964.

Reddy, B. S., Narisawa, T., Maronpot, R., Weisbeurger, J. H. and Wynder, E. L., Animal models for the study of dietary factors and cancer of the large bowel, **Cancer Research**, November 1975, 35(11 part 2), 3421-3426.

Retzlaff, E., Fomtaine, J., and Furuta, W., Effect of daily exercise on life-span of albino rats, **Geriatrics**, March 1966, 21(3), 171-177.

Reynolds, D. K., Nelson, F. L., Personality, life situation , and life expectancy, **Suicide Life Threat Behavior**, Summer 1981 11(2), 99-110.

Ricciuti, H. N., **A review of procedural variations in level of aspiration studies**, Published in San Antonio: Lackland Air Force Base, Human Resources Center, Bulletin 51-24, 1954.

Rickert, W. S. and Forbes, W. F., Changes in collagen with age – VI. Age and smoking related changes in human lung connective tissue, **Experimental Gerontology**, 1976, 11(34), 89-101.

Robertson, J., Brydon, W. G., Tadesse, G., Wenham, P., Walls, A. and Eastwood, M. A., The effect of raw carrot on serum lipids and colon function, **American Journal of Clinical Nutrition**, September 1979, 32(9), 1889-1992.

Rodale, Robert (editor), Low-salting your way to a long life, **Prevention**, May 1982, 6-11.

Rodale, Robert (editor), Quick regeneration for your heart, **Prevention**, July 1983, 9-13.

Ross, M. H. and Bras, G., Lasting influence of early caloric restriction on prevalence of neoplasms in the rat, **Journal of the National Cancer Institute**, November 1971, 47(5), 1095- 1113.

Ross, M. H., Dietary behavior and longevity, **Nutrition Reviews**, October 1977, 35(10), 257-265.

Ross, M. H., Lustbader, E. and Bras, G., Dietary practices and growth responses as predictors of longevity, **Nature**, August 1976, 262(5569), 548-553.

Ross, M. H., Lustbader, E. D. and Bras, G., Dietary practices of early life span and age at death of rats with tumors. **Journal of the National Cancer Institute**, November 1983, 71(5), 947- 954.

Ross, M. H., Nutrition and longevity in experimental animals, **Current Concepts Nutrition**, 1976, 4, 43-57.

Rotter, J. B., Generalized expectancies for internal versus external control of reinforcement, **Psychological Monographs**, 80(1, whole No.609), 1, 966.

Rotter, J. B., Level of aspiration as a method of studying personality Part I. A critical review of methodology, **Psychological Review**, 1942, 49, 463-474.

Rotter J. B., **Social Learning and Clinical Psychology**, Englewood Cliffs, New Jersey: Prentice-Hall, 1954.

Rotter, J. B., Some problems and misconceptions related to the construction of internal vs external control of reinforcement, **Journal of Consulting and Clinical Psychology**, February 1975, 43(1), 56-67.

Rubin, Theodore Isaac, **The Angry Book**, New York, New York: Collier Books, 1969.

Running After 40 by the editors of **Runner's World magazine**, Mountain View, California: Anderson World, Inc., 1980.

Sacher, G. A., Longevity and aging in vertebrate evolution, **Bioscience**, 1978, 28(8), 497-501.

Sapolsky, R. M., Stress and the successful baboon, **Psychology Today**, September 1984, 61-65.

Sauberlich, H. E., Herman, Y. F., Stevens, C. O. and Herman, R. H., Thiamin requirement of the adult human, **American Journal of Clinical Nutrition**, November 1979, 32(11), 2237- 2248.

Schecter, Steve, Winter fasting: mono diets, **Vegetarian Times/Well Being**, January 1982, 33-35.

Scheflen, Albert E. and Scheflen, Alice, **Body Language and Social Order**, Englewood Cliffs, New Jersey: Prentice-Hall, 1972.

Schwartz, A. G., Correlation between species lifespan and capacity to activate 7, 12-dimehylbenz (a) Anthracene to a form mutagenic to a mammalian cell, **Experimental Cell Research**, September 1975, 94(2), 445-447.

Shamberger, R. J., Baughman, F. F., Kalchert, S. L., Willis, C. S. and Hoffman, G. C., Carcinogen-induced chromosomal breakage decreased by antioxidants, **Proceedings of the National Academy of Science**, May 1973, 70(5), 1461-1463.

Shelton, Herbert, M., **Fasting Can Save Your Life**, Bridgeport, Connecticut: Natural Hygiene Press, 1964.

Shostak, Arthur B., **Blue-Collar Stress**, Reading, Massachusetts: Addison-Wesley Publishing Company, 1980.

Shubik, P. and Clayson, D. B., Application of the results of carcinogen bioassays to man, **Archives of Science Publications**, 1976, (13), 241-252.

Shubik, P., Potential carcinogenicity of food additives and contaminants, **Cancer Research**, November 1975, 35(11 Part 2), 3475-3480.

Sinha, Phulgenda, **Yoga Therapy For Common Health Problems**, Washington, D.C.: Yoga Institute, 1976.

Spirduso, W. W., Physical fitness, aging, and psychomotor speed: a review, **Journal of Gerontology**, November 1980, 35(6), 850- 865.

Sitataram, N., Weingartner, H., and Gillin, J. C., Human serial learning: Enhancement with arechloine and choline and impairment with scopolamine, **Science**, July 1978, 201(4352), 274-276.

Smith, F. R., Suskind, R., Thanangkul, O., Leitzmann, C., Goodman, D. S. and Olson, R. E., Plasma vitamin A, retinol-binding protein and prealbumin concentrations in protein-calorie malnutrition. III. Response to varying dietary treatments, **American Journal of Clinical Nutrition**, July 1975, 28(7), 732-738.

Smith, G. S. and Walford, R. L., Influence of the H-2 and H-1 histocompatibility systems upon life span and spontaneous incidences in congenic mice, **Birth Defects**, 1978, 14(1), 281- 312.

Smith, G. S. and Walford, R. L., Influence of the main histocompatibility complex on aging in mice, **Nature**, December 1977, 270(5639), 727-729.

Smith, J. C. Jr., McDaniel, E. G., Fran, F. F. and Halsted, J. A., Zinc: A trace element essential in vitamin A metabolism, **Science**, September 1973, 181(103), 954-955.

Sokoloff, B., Hori, M., Saelhof, C. C., Wrzolek, T. and Imai, T., Aging, atherosclerosis and ascorbic acid metabolism, **Journal of the American Geriatrics Society**, December 1966, 14(12), 1239-1260.

Spanos, E., Barrett, D., MacIntyre, I., Pike, J. W., Safilian, E. F. and Haussler, M. R., Effect of growth hormone on Vitamin D metabolism, **Nature**, May 1978, 273(5659), 246-247.

Spittle, C. R., Atherosclerosis and vitamin C. **Lancet**, June 1972, 1(764), 1335.

Spittle, C., Sporn, M. B. and Newton, D. L., Chemoprevention of cancer with retinoids, **Federation Proceedings**, 38:2528, 1979.

Spritz, N. and Mehkel, M. A., Effects of dietary fats on plasma lipids and lipoproteins: An hypothesis for the lipid lowering effect of unsaturated fatty acids, **Journal of Clinical Investigation**, January 1969, 48(1), 78-86.

Stearn, Jess, **The Power of Alpha-Thinking**, New York, New York: New American Library, 1976.

Stearn, Jess, **Yoga, Youth and Reincarnation**, New York, New York: Bantam Books, 1965.

Stitt, J. T. and Hardy, J. D., Thermoregulation in the squirrel monkey (saimiri sciureus), **Journal of Applied Physiology**, July 1971, 31(1), 48-54.

Stocks, J., Gutteridge, J. M., Sharp, R. J. and Dormandy, T. L., The inhibition of lipid autoxidation by human serum and its relation to serum proteins and alpha-tocopherol, **Clinical Science and Molecular Medicine**, September 1974, 47(3), 223- 233.

Stoltzner, G. H. and Dorsey, B. A., Life-long dietary protein restriction and immune function: response to mitogens and sheep erythrocytes in BALB/C mice, **American Journal of Clinical Nutrition**, June 1980, 33(6), 1264-1271.

Storman, Martin, D., Marital satisfaction variables and female breast cancer patients' predictions of their life expectancies, **Dissertation Abstracts International**, 1982 July Vol. 43(1-B) 266.

Stoyva, Johann (editor), **Biofeedback and Self-Regulation**, New York, New York: Plenum Publishing, 1980.

Stunkard, A. J., Nutrition, aging and obesity: a critical review of a complex relationship. **International Journal of Obesity**, 1983, 7(3), 201-220.

Svoboda, Robert Ayurveda, The art of healing, **Yoga Journal**, November/December 1981, 18-20.

Swami, Rama, Ballantine, Rudolph and Hymes, Alan, **Science Of Breath**, Honesdale, Pennsylvania: The Himalayan International Institute of Yoga Science and Philosophy, 1979.

Syvalahati, E., Lammintausta, R. and Pekkarinen, A., Effect of psychic stress of examination on serum growth hormone, serum insulin, and plasma renin activity, **Acta Pharmacologica et Toxicologica**, April 1976, 38(4), 344-352.

Tagliamonte, A., Fratta, W., Del Fiacco, M. and Gessa, G. L., Possible stimulatory role of brain dopamine in the copulatory behavior of male rats, **Pharmacology and Biochemistry of Behavior**, March/April 1974, 2(2), 257-260.

Takahashi, Y. I., Smith, J. E. and Goodman, D. S., Vitamin A and retinol-binding protein metabolism during fetal development in the rat, **American Journal of Physiology**, October 1977, 233(4), E263-E272.

Tan, N., Biological and medical aspects of ageing, **Nursing Journal of Singapore**, August 1980, 62-65.

Tappel, A.L., Fletcher, B., and Deamer, D., Effect of antioxidants and nutrients on lipid peroxidation fluorescent products and aging parameters in the mouse, **Journal of Gerontology**, October 1973, 28(4), 415-424.

Teevan, Richard C. and Birney, Robert C., (editors), **Theories Of Motivation In Personality and Social Psychology**, Princeton, New Jersey: D. Van Nostrand Company, Inc., 1964.

Thorp, J., Effect of oral contraceptive agents on vitamin and mineral requirements, **Journal of the American Dietetic Association**, June 1980, 76(6), 581-584.

Tinbergen, Nikolaas, Ethology and stress diseases, **Science**, 1974, 185, 20-27.

Tkac, Debora, Selenium, the great protector, **Prevention**, August 1983, 20-22, 24.

Tolmasoff, J. M., Ono, T. and Cutler, R. G., Superoxide dismutase: Correlation with lifespan and specific metabolic rate in primate species, **Proceedings of the National Academy of Science, USA**, May 1980, 77(5), 2777-2781.

Vartabedian, Laurel K., The influence of age difference in marriage on longevity, **Dissertation Abstracts International**, January 1982, 42(7-A), 2934.

Vaughn, Lewis, Cancer update: fighting back with nutrition, **Prevention**, 76-80.

Vaughn, Lewis, Who takes vitamins?, **Prevention**, February 1984, 22-25.

Vir, S. C. and Love, A. H., Vitamin B6 status of the hospitalized aged, **American Journal of Clinical Nutrition**, August 1978, 31(8), 1383-1391.

Vischnudevananda, **The Complete Illustrated Book of YOGA**, New York, New York: Bell Publishing Company, Inc., 1960.

Vkogel, Marata, with Landau, Carolyn and Jannuzzi, Larry, The chemistry of fatigue, **Runner's World**, August 1984, 55-57.

Volicer, L., West, C. and Greene, L., Effect of dietary restriction and stress on body temperature in rats, **Journal of Gerontology**, March 1984, 39(2), 178-182.

Von Esch, P., An inquiry into the effects of a syncretic application of locus of control change techniques to a manpower training program for the economically disadvantaged, Unpublished doctoral dissertation, Boston University, 1978.

Waldron, I., Sex differences in human mortality: the role of genetic factors, **Society of Science Medicine**, 1983, 17(6), 321-333.

Walford, R. L., Immunologic theory of aging: current status, **Federation Proceedings**, September 1974, 33(9), 2020-2027.

Walford, R. L., Liu, R. K., Gerbase, D. M., Mathies, M. and Smith, G. S., Longterm dietary restriction and immune function in mice: response to sheep red blood cells and to mitogenic agents, **Mechanisms of Ageing and Development**, February 1974, 2(6), 447-454.

Walford, Roy L., **Maximum Life Span**, New York, New York: W. W. Norton & Company, 1983.

Walker, A. R., Dietary goals, sensible eating and nutrition in the future, **South African Medical Journal**, January 1980, 57(4), 120-124.

Walker, Norman W., **Become Younger**, Phoenix, Arizona: O'Sullivan Woodside & Company, 1949.

Walker, N. W., **Diet & Salad**, Phoenix, Arizona: O'Sullivan Woodside & Company, 1971.

Walker, N. W., **Raw Vegetable Juices**, New York, New York: The Berkley Publishing Group, 1970.

Wallace, R. K., Physiological effects of transcendental meditation, **Science**, March 1970, 167(926), 1751-1754.

Waltman, R., Tricome, V., Wilson, G. E. Jr., Lewin, A. H., Goldberg, N. L. and Chang, M. M., Volatile fatty acids in vaginal secretions: Human pheromones? **Lancet** September 1973, 2(827), 496.

Warner, D. A. & De Jung, J.E., **Goal Setting Behavior as an Independent Variable Related to the Performance of Educable Mentally Retarded Male Adolescents on Educational Tasks of Varying Difficulty: Final Report** United States Department of Health, Education, and Welfare, Project No. 7-1-115, Washington, D. C. U.S. Government Printing Office, 1969.

Weber, F., Bernard, R. J. and Roy, D., Effects of high-complex- carbohydrate, low-fat diet and daily exercise on individuals 70 years of age and older, **Journal of Gerontology**, March 1983, 38(2), 155-161.

Weindruch, R. H., Cheung, M. K., Verity, M. A. and Walford, R. L., Modification of mitochondrial respiration by aging and dietary restriction, **Mechanisms of Ageing and Development**, April 1980, 12(4), 375-392.

341

Weindruch, R. H., Kristie, J. A., Cheney, K. E., and Walford, R. L., Influence of controlled dietary restriction on immunologic function and aging, **Medical Proceedings**, May 1979, 38(6), 2007-2016.

White, Kristin, Diet & cancer: The real connection, **Vegetarian Times**, September 1984, 23-24, 26.

Williams, H. T., Fenna, D. and Macbeth, R. A., Alpha tocopherol in the treatment of intermittent claudication, **Surgical Gynecology and Obstetrics**, April 1971, 132(4), 662-666.

Wolpe, J., **The Practice of Behavior Therapy**, New York: Pergamon Printers, 1973.

Wolpert, Tom, Nutritional psychology: Is diet the key to psychological health?, **Vegetarian Times**, May 1982, 55-56, 58.

Wood, Ernest, **YOGA**, Harmondsworth, Middlesex, Great Britain; Penguin Books, 1959.

Wood, P.D., Haskell, W., Klein, H., Lewis, S., Stern, M. P. and Farquhar, J. W., The distribution of plasma lipoproteins in middle-aged male runners, **Metabolism**, November 1976, 25(11), 1249-1257.

Woolfolk, R. L., Psychophysiological correlates of meditation, **Archives of General Psychiatry**, October 1975, 32(10), 1326- 1333.

Wozniak, David F., Finger, Stanley, Blumenthal, Herman, Poland, Russell F., Brain damage, stress, and life span: An experimental study, **Journal of Gerontology**, March 1982, 37(2), 161-168.

Wurtman, R. J., Hirsch, M. J. and Growdon, J.H., Lecithin consumption raises serum-free-choline levels, **Lancet**, July 1977, 2(8028), 68-69.

Wurtman, R. J., Rose, C. M., Shou, C. and Larin, F. F., Daily rhythms in the concentrations of various amino acids in human plasma, **New England Journal of Medicine**, July 1968, 279(4), 171-175.

Yeung, D. L., Relationships between cigarette smoking, oral contraceptives, and plasma triglyceride and cholesterol, **American Journal of Clinical Nutrition**, November 1976, 29(11), 1216-1221.

Yogendra, Shri, **Yoga Hygiene Simplified**, New York, New York: Pyramid Books, 1966.

Young, E. A., Nutrition, aging and the aged, **Medical Clinic of North America**, March 1983, 67(2), 295-313. (review)

Zung, W. W. and Giantruco, J. A., Personality dimension and the Self-Rating Depression Scale, **Journal of Clinical Psychology**, April 1971, 27(2), 247-248.

INDEX

Coming soon by the same authors...

METHUSELAH GOURMET COOKBOOK

Cooking to Stay Young, Healthy and Sexy

By

Dr. David C. Gardner

and

Dr. Grace Joely Beatty

This books will bring pleasure to the formidable task of cooking healthy, natural foods that tease the palate of even the most dyed-in-the-wool meat-and-potatoes eater. Recipes have been field-tested and approved by people who do not eat health foods but who consider themselves experts on gourmet cooking. As busy professionals, Joely and David understand the constraints of a pressured schedule and let you in on all of their shortcuts to meal preparation.

If you would like to purchase the book at a 10% prepublication discount, send us your name and address on the coupon below or on a facsimile thereof. When the actual publication date has been determined, you will receive notification of your option to buy at a discount. Please do not send any money at this time.

Name_____

Address_____

City_____

State_____

Zip_____

Yes, please reserve my option to purchase _____ copies of *The Methuselah Gourmet Cookbook* at a 10% prepublication discount.

Mail to: American Training & Research Associates, Inc., Publishers P.O. Box 118, Dept OG, Windham, New Hampshire 03087

CAREER AND VOCATIONAL EDUCATION FOR MILDLY LEARNING HANDICAPPED AND DISADVANTAGED YOUTH

By

DAVID C. GARDNER, GRACE JOELY BEATTY & PAULA L. GARDNER

The authors blend their experience in academia, education and business to produce a unique approach to career and vocational education. They show the reader how to help students acquire technical skills and effective work personalities. The book examines career/vocational program objectives and describes individual assessment and program evaluation. The authors delineate needed curriculum modifications and examine the facts and myths about hiring handicapped and disadvantaged youths. They conclude with information on planning and monitoring individual vocational educational programs and on the future of vocational education.

Published 1984, 222 pages, 27 illustrations, 6 tables
Clothbound-$18.75 (ISBN 0-398-04818-5)

Order through your bookstore or direct from
Charles C Thomas • Publisher
2600 South First Street • Springfield • Illinois • 62717
(217) 789-8980
Sent on approval • Postage paid on MC/Visa/prepaid orders

DISSERTATION PROPOSAL GUIDEBOOK

How to Prepare a Research Proposal and Get It Accepted

By

DAVID C. GARDNER & GRACE JOELY BEATTY

Addressed to anyone facing the formidable task of the dissertation, this volume offers down-to-earth advice on the range of topics pertinent to the first step: the proposal. In the clear prose that characterizes all their writings, Doctors Gardner and Beatty demystify the research proposal process. They explain topic selection, the problem statement, research questions, testable hypotheses, methodology and data analysis. They also provide examples of the various proposal elements and of the different research designs. Tips on how to get the proposal accepted conclude the text.

Published 1980, 112 pages, 3 illustrations, 1 table
Clothbound-$9.50 (ISBN 0-398-04086-9)
Paperbound-$6.75 (ISBN 0-398-04087-7)

Order through your bookstore or direct from
Charles C Thomas • Publisher
2600 South First Street • Springfield • Illinois • 62717
(217) 789-8980
Sent on approval • Postage paid on MC/Visa/prepaid orders

About the Authors

Prominent behavioral scientists
Over 100 professional publications
University professors, licensed psychologists
Consultants to Fortune 500 companies

David C. Gardner, Ed.D., Ph.D., is a licensed psychologist, an Associate Professor at Boston University, and a Principal of American Training and Research Associates, Inc. He served as Chairman of the Department of Business and Career Education at Boston University for five years and as a member of the Board of Directors of the New England Securities Depository Trust Company of the Boston Stock Exchange for two terms. A frequent speaker at national seminars and workshops, he has held marketing and management positions in several Fortune 500 corporations and has appeared on radio and television. He has authored over 100 publications in the behavioral sciences, including four textbooks. Dr. Gardner has specialized in research and teaching on the effective work personality, stress management and the development of methods to help people become more effective. He is listed in "Who's Who in the East" 1981-1982, 1983-1984.

Grace Joely Beatty, Ed.D., Ph.D., is a licensed psychologist and a Principal of American Training and Research Associates, Inc., a consulting firm specializing in market research and organizational change. She is a former Senior Research Associate, Lecturer and Project Manager at Boston University and was an Outstanding Young Woman of America in 1978. Dr. Beatty taught management at the college level for many years and has more than a decade of experience in educational and business psychology. She has specialized in the human factors component of organizational change and minimizing the stressful effects of change on employees. She has also done extensive research on the work personality. A dynamic speaker at national seminars and workshops, Dr. Beatty has authored three textbooks and numerous research articles.